MW00526512

MODERN SOUTHEAST ASIA SERIES

James R. Reckner, *General Editor*

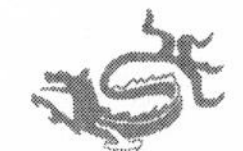

Military Medicine to Win Hearts and Minds

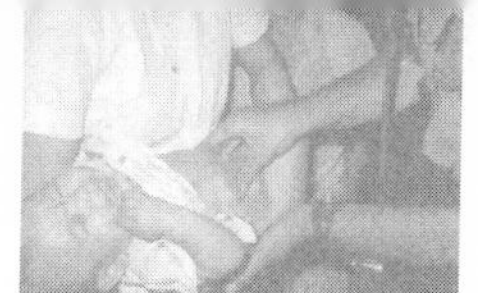

Military Medicine to Win Hearts and Minds

Aid to Civilians in the Vietnam War

Robert J. Wilensky

Texas Tech University Press

This book is typeset in Trump Mediaeval. The paper used in this book meets the minimum requirements of ANSI/NISO Z39.48-1992 (R1997).

Printed in the United States of America

Library of Congress Cataloging-in-Publication Data

Wilensky, Robert J.
Military medicine to win hearts and minds : aid to civilians in the Vietnam War / Robert J. Wilensky.
p. cm. — (Modern Southeast Asia series)
Includes bibliographical references and index.
ISBN 0-89672-532-4 (alk. paper)
1. Vietnamese Conflict, 1961-1975—Medical care. 2. Medical care—Vietnam. I. Title. II. Series.
DS559.44.W53 2004
362.1'0425—dc22
2004002606

04 05 06 07 08 09 10 11 12 / 9 8 7 6 5 4 3 2 1

Texas Tech University Press
Box 41037
Lubbock, Texas 79409-1037 USA
800.832.4042
www.ttup.ttu.edu

To All Who Served in South Vietnam
And Sought to Help the
People of That
Country

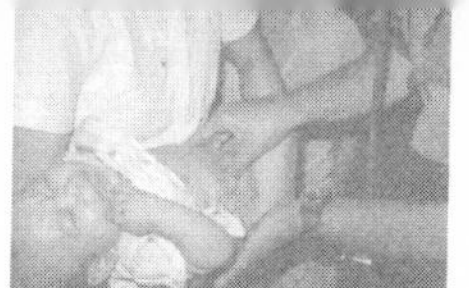

Contents

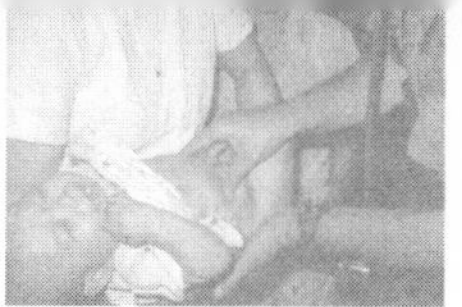

Illustrations

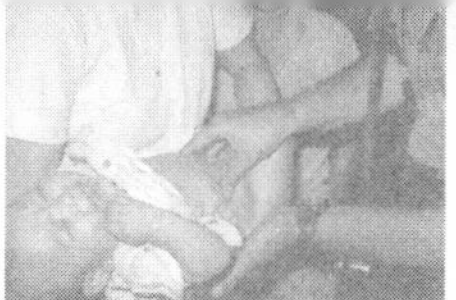

Preface

During 1967 and 1968 I was one of the U.S. military doctors in Vietnam serving in the Army Medical Corps. I spent part of that time caring for civilians in rural areas and orphanages. At that time, I did not realize that it was part of a civic action program to win over the hearts and minds of the Vietnamese civilians.

Even then, I questioned the quality of medical care we were providing. Retrospective doubts about the Vietnam conflict and the programs carried out there abound and should frequently be viewed with a high degree of skepticism. In this instance, however, a document that I wrote in 1968 and uncovered while doing research in the National Archives supports this claim. The lack of diagnostic tools, such as laboratories or X-rays; the absent or irregular patient follow-up; the poor referral system for more advanced care or procedures; and the often-inadequate interpreters were all disturbing. Under direct orders, however, I continued to participate in and carry out the program.

Twenty-five years after my return from Vietnam, I began to study history formally. As with many veterans of that conflict, my interest in it had persisted throughout the years. I realized then that there had never been a comprehensive study of the medical aid programs in Vietnam. The many highly anecdotal reports tended to deal with one location at one time. In part, this was a result of the one-year tour, which applied to medical and support personnel as well as combat troops.

This, then, is my effort to look at the big picture rather than a snapshot of one time or place. I wanted to understand the motivations behind the multiple programs, their evaluations (both by the medical personnel and command), their implementations, and in the long run, their success or failure. My hope is to contribute to an understanding of the use of medical services as an instrument of policy, both to clarify what was done and to provide some insight for the future. If the programs were worthwhile as carried out, then there is justification for continuing to use them in other locales; if they were not, then perhaps manpower and resources should be used in other ways.

No work of many years and significant length is done by the author alone, and this is true in this instance. While I have been engaged in this work over roughly the past seven years, many individuals have freely given me help at various stages. Unfortunately, I cannot recall all their names to list. People in libraries and archives across the country extended themselves on my behalf; many of them did not know me in the least or have any connection to me or my institutions. I greatly appreciate all that they did for me.

Special thanks must go to my friend, teacher, and mentor, Dr. Alan Kraut of The American University in Washington, D.C. He has supported me through this entire endeavor. Others who have been involved since the early years of the project are Dr. Dale Smith of the USUHS and Dr. Anna Nelson of The American University. Extra thanks must go to Dr. Robert J. T. Joy (Col., MC, retired) who has provided both inspiration and guidance.

Fortunately, I can recall the names of two individuals at the National Archives who greatly aided my search for documents and materials: Richard L. Boylan and Jeannine S. Swift. Both of them went beyond their job descriptions to help me and to search diligently in the stacks for what I needed.

Preface

In spite of the many errors I continue to discover, many people have read and commented on the manuscript at various times, helping me to construct proper sentences and put the work in a form that others can read and understand. I thank my daughter, Sara Wilensky, especially in this regard. Eileen Schramm contributed greatly to putting it together in a proper format. I owe a vote of thanks to the outside readers, historians Dr. Jack Shulimson and Dr. Richard A. Hunt. Their suggestions and criticisms have made this a better book.

I must also acknowledge the support I have received from Dr. John Greenwood, Historian, Office of the Surgeon General, and W. T. Gray (Col., MSC, retired) for allowing me the time to leave my other project and work on this one. Dr. Daniel Fox of the Milbank Foundation has been supportive and encouraged me when the work did not seem to be going anywhere.

Lastly, I must thank my wife, Gail R. Wilensky, Ph.D., for her constant support and encouragement, throughout my studies, career change, and time devoted to this project.

Any errors, omissions, or lack of clarity that remains in the work I will claim for myself.

Military Medicine to Win Hearts and Minds

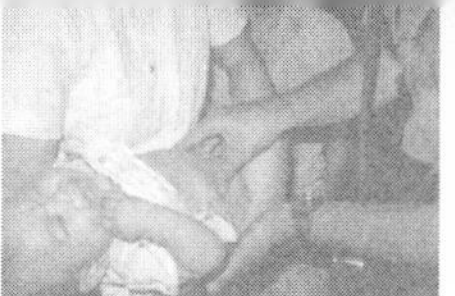

One
Introduction

Young naval lieutenant Dr. Thomas Dooley participated in Operation Passage to Freedom, the massive evacuation of Northern Catholics from North Vietnam to the South following the Geneva Accords of 1954, providing medical care to the refugees both aboard ship and in the camps in South Vietnam.[1] This was the first American military medical activity to aid the civilians of Vietnam. He continued to work in Southeast Asia and was known as *bac si my, bac si Dooley* (American Doctor Dooley). When he and his men passed out medicines, they said, *"La My-Quoc vien-tro"* (This is American aid), to ensure that the people knew it was the United States that was helping them. From that time until the 1973 withdrawal of U.S. military forces from the country, there were multiple programs with American military physicians, nurses, and corpsmen participating in the care of Vietnamese civilians. These programs were based both upon the altruistic inclinations of their participants and the policy aims of the U.S. government.

Medical services have long been an integral part of armies at war, and there is voluminous literature pertaining to the care of injured soldiers, the health of armies, and the role of disease in warfare (see the Bibliographic Essay). The advances in medicine related to war and combat are well documented, as is the application of these advances to peacetime civilian health care. One need only think of our national Emergency Medical Services (EMS) system as an example. The health care of civilians caught in a theater of war has been a neglected subject, as has the provision of civilian medical services as an instrument of policy to aid the war effort. These are the subjects to be examined in this study.

Almost 40 million encounters between American military physicians and Vietnamese civilians occurred from 1963 to 1971 in the Medical Civic Action Program (MEDCAP) alone during the Vietnam conflict.[2] In 1963, almost seven hundred thousand civilians were treated, and this number increased four-fold the next year, reaching a peak of more than 10 million in 1967. Thereafter, as U.S. troops departed, the number of civilians treated rapidly declined (see Appendix A).

From June 1964 through December 1968, there were 69,590 civilians admitted as inpatients to U.S. Army hospitals in South Vietnam, for total bed occupancy of 246,010 days. In addition, 786,472 civilians were treated as outpatients.[3] Aside from questions about motivation for the programs and policy considerations, the sheer volume of this experience, with its associated expense, risks to personnel, and expenditures in time, warrants examination.

There is no previous comprehensive study of the various programs that provided medical care to Vietnamese civilians during the war. This book will examine the motivations for these programs as well as their implementations. It will also try to determine whether the programs were successful in achieving their goals. To do that, it is necessary to define what these goals were. Was the major aim the provision of medical care, or was it, alternatively, the use of the programs to advance the war aims of the administration—that is, the use of medical care as an instrument of policy? In either case, did the programs provide good medical care, and did they contribute to the war effort? Unless the benefits and costs can be determined, no decision regarding the advisability of future efforts in this area can be made.

It is fair to generalize that Americans like to be liked and be praised as humanitarians, even in wartime. The American soldier, sailor, marine, or airman is often portrayed in popular culture giving candy to children by the roadside and doing "good works" in his or her spare time to help the inhabitants of a war-torn region. Providing medical care to orphanages and the infirm is part of this picture, both in reality and in the popular representation. This image of the GI was nurtured in both world wars and in Korea, where the support of the indigenous population was not contested. In Vietnam, however, these activities became part of the campaign to win the support of the people. The question arises whether the altruistic inclinations of those serving abroad constituted a policy and whether it had an impact on how the war was conducted.

In Vietnam, the provision of civilian medical care by military personnel, including physicians and dentists, nurses, and corpsmen, occurred with multiple possible motivations. One possible motivation was pure altruism, the simple desire to help those in need. Another was the use of medicine for strategic purpose, to win "the hearts and minds" of the people.[4] Yet another benefit of treating civilian populations might have been the acquisition of valuable intelligence, both medical and tactical. Medical Corps Col. ElRay Jenkins, when studying the use of medical care for civilian populations at the U.S. Army War College, suggested that the programs could play an important role in countering insurgency.[5] Additional motivations might have included a desire on the part of command to occupy the time of physicians in uniform, as idle military physicians can suffer low morale and become sources of discontent. Gen. William C. Westmoreland ("two-hatted" as both Commander, United States Army, Vietnam [USARV] and Commander, Military Assistance Command, Vietnam [MACV]) thought that medical personnel "are discontented, even feel misused, when they are not occupied in their specialty."[6]

Another important question is whether the goals of the command structure (as opposed to the medical care providers) regarding civilian care were successfully achieved. Did the provision of medical services to civilians contribute to establishing a free and enduring South Vietnam? Further, were the programs primarily intended by command to deliver medical services for humanitarian reasons or to function as an instrument of U.S. policy?

War is complex. No single component functions in a vacuum, but rather various services, such as supply, medical care, and engineering construction, and the fighting branches, such as infantry, armor, and artillery, are all interrelated and dependent on one another. Even so, this study will focus on a single issue—the impact of medical services to civilians and the influence of such medical care on the war effort in Vietnam. To answer the questions posed, some consideration of the concepts of pacification and civic action and the organization of these efforts is required while attempting to place medical services in a proper framework. There was interest at the highest levels in these programs and concern that the Vietnamese peasant be offered as clear alternatives life under the government of Vietnam (GVN) and the Viet Cong (VC).[7] Without an understanding of the civilian/military pacification effort, it is difficult to place medical care to civilians in a proper perspective.

For clarity, it is important to distinguish *civil affairs* from *civic action*, as the two similar terms often appear together in monographs and documents pertaining to Vietnam and can be confusing. *Civil affairs* is the term used to describe the work of the military in providing government services and control in areas under military jurisdiction. Such areas can include friendly territory that is liberated or conquered enemy land.[8] Public health and preventive medicine are components of civil affairs, as the health of an army "parallels the health of the surrounding civilian population."[9] The earliest large-scale venture in this area by the United States occurred during the Mexican-American War. Maj. Gen. Winfield Scott's management of civil affairs was responsible for the Mexican people's opposition to Gen. Santa Anna.[10]

A second term, *civic action*, describes the use of the military to aid the indigenous population.[11] Such aid might include food, clothing, and medical care. Civic action can therefore be a part of civil affairs. The United States was not the first country to adopt military civic action. In his 1950–55 campaign against the Huks, Ramon Magsaysay (defense minister and later president of the Republic of the Philippines) conducted a "program of attraction." Each of his soldiers had two duties: first, to act as an ambassador of goodwill from the government to the people, and second, to kill or capture Huks.[12] This marked the first use of civic action by a modern army against insurgents. The Economic Development Corps Program (EDCOR) grew out of ideas formed during informal discussions between Magsaysay and his American advisor, then Lt. Col. Edward Lansdale, and resulted in the surrender of more Huks than were killed in the campaign.[13] Either Magsaysay, members of his staff, or Lansdale coined the term *civic action.*

The use of military forces to conduct civic action offers several advantages. For very remote and inaccessible areas, the military is often the only government agency equipped and prepared to deliver services. In developing countries, the military is generally more modern and more technically advanced than its counterpart civilian agencies. The military has the additional advantage of being able to provide security for civic action programs when necessary.

A third term to clarify is *pacification*, which basically assures that the rural community will have adequate security to undertake political, social, and economic development.[14] Without adequate security, no significant long-term civic action projects are possible. Participation by the indigenous population does not occur unless and until that population is convinced that their security is assured and the provider, or outside participant, intends to stay for the long term. Further, security must be for twenty-four hours a day, seven days a week, every day and night of the year.

The correlation between rural security and success in pacification cannot be overemphasized. Successful guerilla warfare cannot be conducted in a hostile environment. All pacification programs were aimed at ensuring the support of the people for the GVN. Without that support, ultimately no stable noncommunist government could survive. A guerilla war differs from traditional military operation because its key prize is not control of territory but control of the population.[15] As General Westmoreland stated in his August 1967 report to Adm. Ulysses S. G. Sharp Jr. (Commander in Chief, Pacific [CINCPAC]), "The people's attitude towards the GVN remains in direct proportion to the degree of security afforded them in their hamlets and along lines of communications."[16] In Vietnam, the real battle was to win the support of the people for the government.

Unlike conventional wars, the war in Vietnam lacked the ordinary criteria to judge success or failure on particular decisions and operations. There were no front lines to mark advances or retreats. Comparison of casualties was approximate and suspect. Wounded or killed were routinely removed from the battlefields by both sides. While popular support is an important indicator of success, it was difficult to measure in Vietnam. In the hamlets, both sides maintained a constant presence. Saigon controlled much of the country in the daytime; the VC dominated a large part of the same population at night. "For the villagers, the presence of the Government during the day had to be weighed against its absence after dark, when Saigon's cadres almost invariably withdrew into the district or provincial capitals."[17] These same factors complicate the evaluation of medical aid programs and force greater reliance on impressionistic evidence and anecdotal data rather than hard data and statistical analysis. As former Secretary of State Henry Kissinger concluded, to be effective, the pacification program had to meet two conditions: (1) it had to provide security for the population, and (2) it had to establish a political and institutional link between the villages and Saigon. Neither condition was ever met.[18]

This study will begin with a brief examination of previous civilian care by the U.S. government. These precedents of the use of military medicine in conflicts before Vietnam will be examined for degree of involvement, motives, and effectiveness. Disease has frequently incapacitated more soldiers than combat, and troops serving within an area of poor sanitation and widespread disease are at great risk. Particular attention will be paid to whether these services were provided primarily to protect the U.S. military personnel stationed within the area or to benefit the indigenous population. Both of these could, of course, occur simultaneously, but the question is which was the prime motivation for the program.

In discussing the various medical aid programs, the nature of the conflict in Vietnam must be borne in mind. In an unconventional war without front lines or protected rear areas, all personnel, including medical, in the theater are at risk. Sending small groups into the population obviously increases these risks. The first American serviceman killed in Vietnam on 22 December 1961, Sp4c. James T. Davis, was a combat medic.[19] At least twenty-one military physicians were killed in Southeast Asia by January 1972, though it is unclear whether some of the aircraft accidents (primarily of helicopters) were due to hostile action.[20] Maj. Charles L. Kelly, MSC, the third commander of the 57th Medical Detachment, established the "dustoff" system. In fact, "Dustoff" was his call sign. He was killed while attempting to evacuate wounded soldiers on 1 July 1964, the 149th American, and the first medical evacuation pilot, to die in Vietnam.[21] Ninety commissioned and warrant officers were killed in Vietnam flying medical evacuation helicopters, and another 380 pilots were wounded or injured.[22]

The first army doctor to lose his life in Vietnam, Capt. Thomas W. Stasko, MC, was killed in a helicopter crash near Saigon on 18 February 1966.[23] Rocket and mortar fire from a distance strikes randomly. The commanding officer of the 45th Surgical Hospital in Tay Ninh, Maj. Gary P. Wratten, MC, was killed in a mortar attack in November 1966.[24]

While serving at the 312th Evacuation Hospital, 1st Lt. Sharon A. Lane was the first nurse killed in Vietnam.[25] She was the only nurse to die from direct enemy action. At least eight nurses died in Vietnam, and one died of a disease contracted in Vietnam after being medevaced to Japan.[26] After the 1968 Tet battle, the danger involved in MEDCAP missions was so great that army nurse Maj. Marguarite J. Rossi at the 2nd Surgical Hospital in Chu Lai maintained that the "combat and social welfare roles should not coexist."[27]

With good reason, physicians constantly worried about their own physical safety. Special Forces (SF) medical teams on occasion had to "buy" their way out of confrontation with the guerillas by giving them medical supplies.[28] The 173rd Airborne Brigade reported four fatalities that occurred during a medical team's return visit on the MEDCAP when a claymore mine was detonated in the building where they treated patients. None of the villagers warned them.[29] In another instance, a physician from the 93rd Evacuation Hospital in Long Binh found an unexploded claymore mine in the village square where they were holding the MEDCAP. The air force aid station personnel at Nha Trang reported being stripped clean of medical supplies when they were overrun during a MEDCAP mission in a nearby hamlet. Thereafter, the unit discontinued MEDCAP. Further, fear of ambushes served to limit scheduled return visits to a dispensary or hamlet, which is important in regard to follow-up medical care. Whether these fears were justified is less significant than the effect that they generated on the programs.

Numerous senior government officials identified medical care to the civilian population as an essential tool of foreign policy in the battle to win Vietnamese hearts and minds. Medical Corps Brig. Gen. James H. Forcee recognized medical care as an instrument that could both "do good" and gain political influence in 1961.[30] Surgeon General Leonard B. Heaton, however, underscored the political character of the medical efforts when he said, "It is not truly a military responsibility to care for the civilian population of Vietnam."[31] In 1963, ambassador to Vietnam Henry Cabot Lodge stated that medicine was the "best media for the people-to-people program."[32] Secretary of the Army Cyrus Vance went so far as to suggest that teaching and assistance programs staffed by off-duty personnel were more important than the treatment of Vietnamese and American personnel in hospitals.[33] In his *1968 Report on the War in Vietnam,* General Westmoreland stated, "Among the many Civic Action projects undertaken in Vietnam, perhaps none had a more immediate and dramatic effect than the Medical Civic Action Program." Nearly a decade later, Col. Bedford H. Berrey, while in the Office of the Assistant Secretary of Defense, wrote that "medicine deserved recognition as an active partner of American foreign policy."[34]

How military commanders perceived the proper role of their medical personnel determined how medical services were delivered and whether a long lasting program of benefit persisted. The army medical service was certainly used as an instrument of goodwill and consciously exploited to further the accomplishment of the army's mission.[35] Despite the voluminous writing on the Vietnam conflict, there is little commentary in the secondary literature regarding the role of medical care of the civilian population in winning the hearts and minds of the peasantry, even in those works focusing on pacification programs.

Analyses generated by the military focus on medical care of the wounded soldier. There is only brief mention of civilian care, with minimal discussion of policy implications. While recent shorter papers originating within the military explore this topic to a degree, they all lack a full discussion of policy decision making, implementation, and evaluation of the programs, including the potential effectiveness of similar programs in the future. This is also true in works describing allied efforts in Vietnam.

An important question to consider is whether the delivery of medical care was intended to reflect positively on the United States or on the host government that the United States supported. Who benefits by attempts to win the hearts and minds of the people? Can the delivery of medical care by U.S. soldiers gain goodwill that is transferred to the host government, or does that goodwill simply stay with the U.S. "foreign" troops? Lt. Gen. Leonard D. Heaton, Surgeon General of the Army, was adamant that medical people remain in uniform and not wear civilian clothes.[36] If the goodwill stayed with the U.S. medical personnel in Vietnam, did the programs actually make a difference and facilitate implementing American policy? The various programs had different components of direct delivery of medical care, consultation with Vietnamese health providers of all types, and teaching Western medicine. An instructional program is long lasting but less dramatic. It might have less immediate effect on the population one is attempting to win over, but in the long run, it might have more medical benefit and has the potential to be of lasting impact.

Another previously mentioned aspect of the MEDCAP program was the opportunity to gather medical intelligence, which has multiple facets. Medical intelligence can inform about the enemy presence by disclosing diseases or forms of diseases in the population that are not normally seen in an area. An enemy's condition is revealed by the degree of sophistication of their medical care and supplies. Moreover, the origin of these supplies can give clues about outside support for the enemy. Medical teams working with the indigenous population can discern attitudes among the people that are hidden from combat arms and intelligence personnel. If the people trust and like the medical personnel, they might warn of possible enemy attacks in advance, thus providing tactical intelligence through medical channels. This actually happened on more than one occasion in Vietnam.

Physician, nurse, and medic memoirs and diaries provide an incomplete record of the programs. Limited by the one-year tour time frame, such narratives tend to be highly anecdotal and devoid of policy analysis. They also tend to suffer from a very restricted perspective, both geographically and temporally. They report what happened in one place at one time. There is no previous work that looks at the various programs over time and space, rather than snapshots of singular occurrences that might hold true for the entire conflict. This study seeks to remedy that deficiency.

As in any conflict, examination of one component, facet, or program in Vietnam does not offer a complete picture unless it is related to the whole. Medical services paralleled the course of the war in many ways: early on they were sparse, with the buildup of troop strength they increased, and then they were withdrawn as the American troop pull-out occurred. The ability to provide services to the civilians and the use of these services to advance policy aims increased as the troop levels reached their maximum in 1969 and declined as troops were withdrawn. Medical services were withdrawn in proportion to the fighting forces and other support units.

American personnel had been involved in Vietnam from the waning years of World War II. Office of Strategic Services (OSS) members were in contact with the Viet Minh and Ho Chi Minh, who were fighting the Japanese, primarily to aid downed American flyers. These contacts continued for a short time after the war was over during the period when Ho Chi Minh declared Vietnamese independence and sought American recognition.

Whereas President Roosevelt had strongly opposed reinstitution of French colonial rule in Southeast Asia,[37] President Truman reversed this policy under the pressures of the Cold War. French support in Europe was needed for a successful containment policy, and the price for that support in Europe was support, or at least acquiescence to, a return of French control in Indochina. In 1949 and 1950, Mao Tse Tung and the Communists gained control over all of mainland China, the Soviet Union exploded its first atomic bomb, and China and the USSR recognized the government of Ho Chi Minh. The United States considered this recognition as evidence that Ho Chi Minh had always intended to establish a communist regime in Vietnam.

In February 1950, the French requested assistance in Indochina. President Truman received NSC 68, which put forth the containment policy in April and the next month announced that the United States would aid the French in Vietnam. War broke out in Korea in June 1950, and by the time that conflict ended in 1953, the United States was subsidizing about 80 percent of the French costs in Vietnam.

The French war in Indochina, sometimes referred to as the First Indo-Chinese War, went badly, culminating in the defeat at Dien Bien Phu in 1954. This military defeat coincided with the Geneva Conference on Indochina and had significant impact on the nature of the Geneva Accords of 1954. The United States was not a signatory to those accords, but it "took note" of them and declared it would "refrain from the threat or the use of force to disturb them." Vietnam was split into two temporary regroupment zones at the seventeenth parallel, with the anticipation of reunification elections in 1956. Elections were never held, as Prime Minister Ngo Dinh Diem maintained they would not be conducted fairly in the North. The United States did not press the matter, as most high-ranking American authorities realized that if the elections were held, Ho Chi Minh would win. President Dwight D. Eisenhower pledged economic and military assistance to Prime Minister Diem in South Vietnam.

In 1959 Viet Minh regroupees—southerners who had gone north during the 300-day regroupment period following the signing of the Geneva Accords in 1954 when there was supposed to be free movement between the two parts of the country—began to reinfiltrate into South Vietnam to join the "stay behind" cadres and form the VC. As the insurgency gained momentum, the government of North Vietnam made a decision to support the military overthrow of the Diem regime. President Eisenhower pledged increased military aid to the Republic of Vietnam on 5 May 1960; and in December 1960, the National Liberation Front (NLF), the political arm of the VC, announced its existence. Direct participation of U.S. Civil Affairs personnel in the counterinsurgency began in 1960.[38] In June 1961, the United States agreed to increase the Military Assistance Advisory Group (MAAG) beyond the 658-man level, which had been approved by the International Control Commission in late 1960. This was done as the war was being lost in the fall of 1961.[39]

The American ambassadors in Saigon, Henry Cabot Lodge, Jr., (on his first of two tours of duty as ambassador) and his successor, retired Gen. Maxwell Taylor, advised against a large American land force. Both feared the needs of even a small combat force would require insertion of increasingly large numbers of troops. Both Taylor and Secretary of Defense Robert McNamara, however, predicted in 1961 that U.S. troops would be needed to preserve the Saigon government.[40] In December 1961, two army helicopter companies arrived in Republic of Vietnam (RVN) to bolster the Army, Republic of Vietnam (ARVN), and by the end of 1961, U.S. troop strength was slightly over four thousand men.[41] The MACV was formed in January 1962 with Gen. Paul D. Harkins as its commander.

U.S. forces in Vietnam before the military buildup of 1965 were limited. Troops under President Kennedy totaled about twenty-five thousand,[42] with most being advisors. The January 1963 Battle of Ap Bac showed that an NLF guerilla force could successfully fight against a multibattalion ARVN force supported only by U.S. helicopters and artillery.[43] Ap Bac revealed the VC's strength as well as the ARVN's inefficiency. Adding substantial U.S. ground forces required careful consideration of the political climate.

Journalist Stanley Karnow suggests that by participating in the

November 1963 overthrow of Ngo Dinh Diem and his brother Ngo Dinh Nhu and their resulting deaths, the United States assumed a responsibility for Vietnam that would lead inevitably to the entry of American combat troops.[44] With the assassination of President Kennedy later that month, President Lyndon Johnson was forced to choose whether to continue Kennedy's program or withdraw. President Johnson chose to continue to support the South Vietnamese. For a year and a half, short-lived military dictatorships and governments followed in rapid succession, and South Vietnam "wallowed in political confusion."[45] Paradoxically, the American intervention weakened the South Vietnamese by creating a "crippling sense of dependency among Saigon officials" on the Americans and lulling them into believing that the United States would never leave South Vietnam.[46]

Harkins was replaced by Gen. William C. Westmoreland in June 1964. That same month, Ambassador Taylor replaced Ambassador Lodge. In August 1964, the reported attacks on U.S. naval ships in the Gulf of Tonkin occurred. The attacks provided an excuse for the congressional Gulf of Tonkin Resolution, which both Presidents Johnson and Nixon relied on as the legal authorization to conduct the war. No definitive combat operations were begun at that time, as the presidential election of 1964 was pending.

In February 1965, the Rolling Thunder bombing campaign of North Vietnam was started to show the North Vietnamese that the United States would support the South and to shore up the South Vietnamese government. In March 1965, American marine units landed in Da Nang to provide support and protection for air force units but quickly were authorized to conduct offensive operations. Army combat units soon followed, and the predictions of Taylor and McNamara that additional troops would be required were fulfilled. Medical units were inserted along with other support forces.

Two

Previous Use of Medical Care for Foreign Civilians

The Vietnam conflict was not the first use of military medical care of civilians, nor was the United States the only country to employ medical services in the effort to win over the population. For the provision of medical services to be effective as an instrument of policy, certain conditions, such as a lack of medical care for the civilians and a civilian population whose support was sought by both sides in the conflict, needed to exist. On some occasions, the need to provide medical services began to protect the troops, as soldiers are at risk from diseases within the surrounding population.

The creation of the Merchant Marine, around the time of the nation's founding, brought with it a need to provide its sea-going members with medical care. This ultimately led to the present-day United States Public Health Service (USPHS), which was established by an act of Congress in 1798.[1] Marine hospitals and physicians were authorized to assist local governments in combating epidemics of cholera and yellow fever. The present mission of the USPHS is to promote and protect the health of the civilian population.[2]

Within the United States, the military provided medical care to civilians during the American Civil War, the first time this practice had occurred. In that instance, the motivation was really necessity, as the freedmen gathered around the Union army bases and constituted a real potential source of disease. Any army is vulnerable to disease present within its own environment.[3] If there are no civilian caretakers, then the military must provide the care for its own protection. The freedmen, or former slaves, had previously had their medical care, clothing, and food provided by their masters. This circumstance ended with Union army victories or when the slaves fled from bondage. In this instance, care of the civilians was not intended to win their support in the conflict, as the Union forces already had their support. It was an example of defensive medicine.

The Freedmen's Bureau was established 3 March 1865. Even though a Union army major general, Oliver O. Howard, commanded the bureau, it was not a purely military organization. Instead, it functioned alongside the army as a health and welfare provider. It was, therefore, an early example of the blurring of lines between the military and civilian worlds in providing care for civilians. The bureau offered both short-term services to provide medical aid and also established long-term programs such as the first medical schools for African Americans. These responsibilities continued throughout the early years of Reconstruction.[4] The Howard University School of Medicine, created by the bureau in 1867, remains to this day the most highly regarded institution devoted to the medical education of African Americans.

The role of military medical services in nonconventional warfare, as in the Philippines or Vietnam, may well differ from that in conventional wars. While the primary mission of preserving the fighting strength is unchanged, secondary activities of the medical corps in combating guerillas and insurgency conflicts expand and become increasingly important. The need to win the hearts and minds of the populace does not exist when the army only seeks to repel an invader (as in both world wars and Korea), but is of paramount importance in counterinsurgency warfare.

This then is the first criterion for the use of military medical services as an instrument or tool of policy: the support of the people must be sought and fought over by both sides in the conflict. If one side has that support, or, to put it another way, if one side has no hope of gaining that support as in the German invasions of France, then whether there is any provision of medical care for the people will be irrelevant. They will never be won over to support the hated invaders.

An example of this occurred during the Spanish-American War of 1898 in both Cuba and later in the Philippines during the post-war insurrection. After the defeat of Spain, Filipino insurgents, who had anticipated independence in the wake of the defeat of Spain, carried on the war utilizing guerilla tactics. Pacification became a major component of military strategy.[5] Medical assistance was a part of the campaign to win over the civilian population. Direct care was rendered to civilians, with a focus on preventive medicine and an extensive public health program was begun. The army instituted extensive vaccination programs against smallpox, programs to eliminate bubonic plague, and measures to ensure a safe water supply.[6] Lt. Gen. Arthur MacArthur felt that medical care was significant in winning over the urban civilian population, depriving the guerillas of their support base and supplies necessary to continue the fight and securing victory.[7] Thus, the provision of medical care to the indigenous civilians was utilized as an instrument or tool of policy. While both historians Mary Gillette in her official history of the late nineteenth- and early twentieth-century medical department[8] and John Morgan Gates in his history of the U.S. Army in the Philippines[9] noted the significance of health programs to the military success in the Philippines, and Franklin Kemp and William Lyster discussed military physicians providing care for civilians in contemporaneous writings,[10] none remarked upon it as a policy tool.

U.S. authorities on occasion ignored cultural, economic, and other practical aspects of the health problems. Health practices advocated and enforced by the U.S. troops often conflicted with long held cultural habits and traditions. In the rural Philippines, livestock and pigs roamed freely in the villages, often living below elevated houses. Coercion was occasionally needed to carry out sanitation programs,[11] as in the cholera eradication efforts in Balangiga. The medical problems associated with prostitution were due in part to the dependency on U.S. dollars created by the war and not simply a disease or public health problem;[12] however, U.S. authorities chose not to address that portion of the problem. Most soldiers disliked pacification work as it was difficult and unrewarding, and they found the political aspect of it especially unappealing.[13]

Another aspect of the medical program arose in the Philippines. Gillette remarked on what might have been the first use of the United States' medical service for intelligence purposes, "in at least some instances they (the medical officers) may have been involved in extracting information from captured Filipinos."[14] Participating in the torture of captives, even to ensure that they survived, still violates basic medical ethics. Captured medical supplies provided an evaluation of the state of the enemy, another aspect of medical intelligence.

The second criterion for military medical care of civilians to be significant in the war effort also existed in the Philippines: there was a deficiency in available medical care. It is almost self-evident that supplying a commodity or service that is already present in abundance will not influence the feelings of the people. During the two world wars, Western medical systems of care existed in France, for example, even though the wars caused shortages of materials and personnel. Therefore, the provision of these services would not win over the people, if that had been necessary. Providing humanitarian aid to these civilians was laudable, but it did not significantly contribute to the war effort.

The Pacific Theater of operations in World War II provided a similar model. There was no need to win over the civilians. As the island hopping campaign proceeded toward the Japanese homeland, the indigenous populations rejoiced to be rid of the invaders. Further, once an island had been liberated, it was no longer significant in the conflict as in no instance was an island retaken by the Japanese. After expelling the Japanese from each island, islanders were left to rebuild their communities. Any allied efforts to improve medical services were not vital to the war effort.

In post-war Japan, Gen. Douglas MacArthur, who had acted as aide to Gen. Leonard Wood in Washington (1911) and the Philippines (1921), instituted medical programs of immunizations, established health centers, and promoted preventive medicine programs. These medical programs literally reached every citizen of Japan and were part of the civil affairs program. As post-war assistance, they contributed to the recovery of Japan and to goodwill between the citizens of Japan and the United States.[15]

At the end of World War II, most of the doctors and nurses in Korea were Japanese and returned to Japan.[16] In the late 1940s, selected Korean military medical personnel began training with U.S. Army medical units located in South Korea. With the assistance of U.S. military medical personnel, a Korean Army Medical School was opened in 1949. The Korean Army Medical Field Service School was staffed by instructors from the U.S. Medical Field Service School in San Antonio, Texas. In 1950, the U.S. Department of the Army allocated a number of spaces for Republic of Korea (ROK) personnel to train in American medical schools. All these actions occurred before the outbreak of hostilities on the Korean peninsula.[17]

With the swift invasion by the North Koreans, Seoul was quickly overrun at the start of the war. The Communists captured medical personnel who had been largely concentrated in the capital. Medical and welfare supplies were taken along with the personnel. Fortunately, the rehabilitation of the Japanese pharmaceutical and medical supply industries by the United States at the end of World War II had created a nearby source for the replacement of these vital items in Korea.[18]

In many ways, the Korean War was similar to the European Wars, especially after China entered the conflict. There was a front line that shifted geographically with the fortunes of war. Medical services suffered greatly due to the war, but military medicine was not needed to gain the support of the indigenous population who viewed the enemy as invaders to be expelled. In addition to providing medical service to its own forces while halting the invasion of the Republic of Korea, the U.S. Army assisted the ROK Army with its medical services in a technical advisory, medical supply, and medical equipment capacity. During periods of relative quiet, U.S. medical personnel assisted many civilians and civilian agencies in Korea.[19]

The major medical civic action activity in Korea occurred following cessation of hostilities. The Armed Forces Assistance to Korea (AFAK) program was carried out from 1953 to 1970.[20] It was Medical Corps Col. Wallis Craddock's belief that, while the U.S. military succeeded in halting Communist aggression on the peninsula, the lasting friendship of the Korean people stemmed from the medical aid program, not military achievement.[21] This viewpoint is perhaps not surprising coming from a member of the Medical Corps. While this is highly desirable from a standpoint of national policy, it is very different from using medical services during the conflict to aid in achieving victory.

Both the indigenous medical care system and the type of warfare in Vietnam differed greatly from the pattern of the world wars or the Korean conflict. There was no single or shifting front line but rather a series of simultaneously occurring enclaves. The same territory was contested repeatedly, and the civilians were subjected to pressure and influence from both sides. Major civic action and pacification efforts, including medical care services, were utilized to garner Vietnamese support.[22]

World Wars I and II and the Korean conflict were conventional conflicts, in that there was a relatively well defined but changing front line. The aim was to expel an invader. The U.S. leadership initially viewed the Vietnam conflict as an insurrection by the southern-based VC instigated, supported, and directed by North Vietnam. Much of this support and the infiltration of People's Army of Vietnam (PAVN) troops occurred via the Ho Chi Minh Trail in eastern Laos and Cambodia.[23] While there were certainly North Vietnamese troops fighting in South Vietnam from very early on, with PAVN forces entering South Vietnam in 1964 and 1965, and North Vietnamese troops repeatedly attempting to infiltrate the Demilitarized Zone (DMZ), a successful conventional invasion across the border did not occur until U.S. withdrawal was virtually complete. At that time, no civic action of any kind would have affected the ultimate outcome. In retrospect, there was always a greater military involvement by North Vietnam than the U.S. leadership recognized, while the initiation of the conflict was due to those in the South to a greater extent than the United States chose to acknowledge. It is conceivable that no civic action programs could have the degree of impact on the outcome of the war that was intended.

While the focus of this work is on U.S. actions during the Vietnam conflict, it is important to note that other countries also engaged in the use of medical services as part of their civic action programs. For example, in the early years of World War II, Finnish army doctors were sent to treat the peasants in remote Karelian villages. They delivered medicines and food. As a result, "there were people willing to run for miles across deep snow to the nearest Finnish Army post to give alarm whenever the Soviet raiders came."[24] Also during World War II, the Japanese opened two small hospitals in Hanoi and Saigon for Vietnamese civilians. According to historian David G. Marr, "Gifts of medicine, food, and money from the [Japanese] home islands to ill or injured Vietnamese received wide publicity."[25] It was an eerie foreshadowing of the American experience. Medical services were also utilized to win over the "native" populations in North Africa during the European colonization of that region, as well as in India during the period of the Raj.[26] While these experiences differ somewhat from the use of medicine as a tool during a full-scale war, they are examples of the use of medicine and especially military medicine as an instrument of policy.

In 1962, President Kennedy developed a plan to aid emerging nations in utilizing military civic action to contribute to economic and social development in their countries. In January 1962 NSAM 124 (National Security Action Memorandum) established a new interagency group, chaired by Maxwell Taylor to coordinate the "subterranean war"—the task of the Special Group (Counterinsurgency) was ensuring "the use of U.S. resources with maximum effectiveness in preventing and resisting subversive insurgency in friendly countries."[27] It was implemented in Latin America, Ethiopia, and elsewhere in Asia, as well as in Vietnam.[28] A major problem with the program was that it was imposed on the military, rather than arising from within it.[29] The medical portion of this plan, which would become part of the counterinsurgency program, focused on health and sanitation needs.[30]

The use of military forces to conduct civic action offers several advantages. For very remote and inaccessible areas, the military forces are often the only government agency equipped and prepared to deliver services. In developing countries, the military is generally more modern and more technically advanced than its counterpart civilian agencies.[31] The military has the additional advantage of being able to provide security for civic action programs when necessary.

Chapters 3 and 4 will examine first the early U.S. military endeavors in Vietnam and the less formalized medical assistance programs and then the more formal and structured programs during and after the major American troop buildup of 1965. Chapter

5 will undertake a medical evaluation of the various programs, and Chapter 6 will look at them as a policy tool. The final chapter will draw conclusions from the preceding chapters and make some suggestions as to how best to use medicine as an instrument of policy in the future.

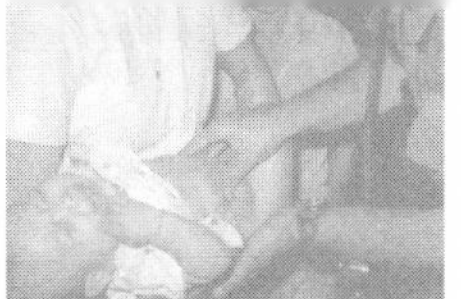

Three
The Ad Hoc or Informal Programs

During the early years of American military involvement in Vietnam under the MAAG, there were few troops in country, and they were organized as small units operating relatively independently. The provision of medical care by these units was part of their mission as a part of civic action programs. It was carried out in a rather informal nonregimented manner. This was true until the large troop buildup of 1965 that occurred under the control of the new command, the MACV. A brief discussion of the status of medicine in Vietnam will clarify the situation the Americans found when they entered the country.

The pressing need for medical care in Vietnam provided the opportunity for medical aid programs to be effective. Thus, one of the necessary criterions was fulfilled. Vietnam had not developed a modern science based, nationwide health care system as of the 1960s. South Vietnam had only 1,400 physicians, 1,000 of whom were in its army. Even though many physicians serving in the army also had civilian practices, there were only four hundred nonmilitary physicians to care for 16 million civilians. Almost all nonmilitary physicians were located in the major cities of Saigon, Da Nang, and Hue.[1] This pattern was not going to change in the near future. Out of the 174 students in their final year at the medical school in Saigon, only the fourteen women were not scheduled to be drafted for four years of military service.[2] Since most nurses were men, the draft and compulsory military service depleted civilian nursing ranks, creating a severe shortage of nurses as well.[3]

Vietnam and the conflict there thus constituted an excellent opportunity to investigate military care of civilians in wartime. The civilian population was strongly courted by all participants in the conflict. All parts of the country were in dispute virtually all of the time. Both sides realized that victory could not be achieved without winning the support of the peasantry in this rural society.

The introduction of modern medicine into remote rural areas was accompanied by problems of communication greater than language barriers. Also, there were many different cultural groups in Southeast Asia, each with their own traditions and mores. Vietnamese medicine could be Sino-Vietnamese, the medicine of the North (*thuôc Bac*), or Vietnamese proper, also called Annamite medicine or the medicine of the South (*thuôc Nam*). In the 1960s, there were about 4,600 practitioners of Chinese traditional medicine (*ong lang*) in Vietnam, six hundred of whom lived in Saigon. Unlike other practitioners, sorcerers, found among the Montagnard (mountain people) tribes, relied on spirits and incantations. These healers provided much of the health care in the villages and hamlets.[4] Folk remedies such as cupping and pinching to raise a welt or cause a bruise were widely used.

The Vietnamese, as do all people, desired good health, and they respected methods that work, though they first required a demonstration. The desire for health is not the same thing as desiring medical care, however. When sick or injured, there is an acceptance of medical care to regain health. There is a Vietnamese proverb: "Look at the old, and learn the new" (*Ôn gô tri tân*). Clearly, the Vietnamese had some attitudes regarding medicine that Americans did not share or easily understand.

The lack of environmental sanitation was probably the most significant health problem in Vietnam during the war. Garbage disposal was primitive and collection practices were haphazard in the big cities. This contributed to the large fly and rodent populations and the endemic presence of plague. Plague, known to South Vietnam since 1906, became a major epidemiological problem in 1963 and increased in severity throughout the war due to refugee overcrowding and poor sanitation.[5] South Vietnam had been a rural country, with almost 90 percent of the population living in the villages and hamlets before the war. With the insecurity caused by the war, there was a massive relocation of the population into the urban centers, which held almost half of the people by the war's end. Even when trying to improve sanitation systems, it was necessary to be aware of local practices and customs. In one instance, a well was dug by the Special Forces (SF) troops to aid an unnamed hamlet in the Central Highlands. It was in an area away from animals and uncontaminated. The pump kept breaking. Ultimately, it was learned that the old well was under the supervision of the Buddhist Bonze (monk), and a fee or offering was made when water was drawn from that well. Since the Buddhists had not been consulted about the new well, they had lost face or "merit" as termed by the Buddhists. After this situation was corrected and the administration of the new well was transferred to the monks, there was a sudden cessation in the downtime of the well.[6]

Polio was endemic throughout Vietnam. Oral polio vaccine was not used in the outlying provinces. The reason for this demonstrated both the conditions of the rural economy and the rural health care situation. Oral polio vaccine was not used because in the rural provincial hospitals there was no electricity and, therefore, no refrigeration, which was necessary to preserve the vaccine.[7] Changing to a Western medical system required changes in the economy, the infrastructure, and the culture as well as medical education.

Life in rural Vietnam revolved around the family, the village, religion, and crops.[8] As many had never gone more than twenty or thirty miles from home, they often feared the town or city and were reluctant to go to the hospital. There was a fear of the world outside of the village; patients told they required hospitalization occasionally disappeared.[9]

Major decisions, including those regarding medical treatment, were made only after consultation within the family in rural Vietnam. While one family member frequently accompanied the patient to the hospital, there might have been times when an entire family would do so.[10] This tradition made transporting the patient complicated and created crowding and disruption at the hospital.

Since a family often slept two or more to a bed at home, many patients were unwilling to stay in a hospital without a family member. Parents might have demanded to stay in the same bed with a sick child so that he or she would not be afraid.[11] When American politicians or investigators visited Vietnamese hospitals, they almost uniformly commented on the fact that there were two or three patients in a bed. They did not understand that this was normal and most comfortable for the Vietnamese, who often were uncomfortable if made to stay in a bed alone. It did not mean there were inadequate beds available.

Most Vietnamese people attached great importance to dying at home and being buried near the village. Many villages prohibit the transportation of corpses. Therefore, when a patient is critically ill or worsens in the hospital, his family might take him home to be near the home burial ground.[12] It is better to die at home than to take a chance on getting well but dying far away. This tradition of ancestor worship and the strong desire to be near familial burial grounds also contributed to unhappiness with the various relocation programs, such as the strategic hamlet program, that were attempted as pacification measures. Leaving ancestral burial grounds went against the strong familial obligations and destroyed relationships within the family of father to ancestors, sons to fathers, younger to older sons.

French policy had been to limit Vietnamese training to basic areas, retaining specialist skills for the French practitioners.[13] This was analogous to the French civil service system, which limited the Vietnamese they trained to relatively low-level positions, retaining the policy and decision-making jobs for the French. The French never had any intention of preparing the Vietnamese for self-government.[14]

Deficiencies in the number and training of medical personnel other than physicians were significant. In 1956, the United States Agency for International Development (USAID) sponsored a program to improve government nursing training and midwifery services. There had been an acute shortage of nurses. The facilities for training nurses were limited, and the low pay schedules for nurses caused many trained in the field to leave it for other more remunerative opportunities.[15] Before the training programs instituted by the U.S. agencies, virtually all the nurses in Vietnam had been men. The Minister of Health began to encourage women to enter nursing. The medical community initially threatened female nurses and called them "harlots" but eventually accepted them. By the time of the 1968 Tet Offensive, most of the nurse trainees were female and, therefore, exempt from the draft.[16]

The concept of nursing care differed greatly from that in the United States. In Vietnam, the patient's family was responsible for providing nursing care and food in the hospital. Often, families would cook meals on a charcoal or gas burner at the patient's bedside. Medical Corps Capt. Ralph Levin discussed the nurses at the Quang Tin Province Hospital in his end-of-tour report. Their backgrounds ranged from no formal training to four years in nursing school. According to Levin, nurses failed to accurately record routine vital signs, such as temperatures and blood pressures, or carry out physicians' orders, which he described as "disappointing." The situation worsened on weekends when patients did not receive their medications, and no notes were made on the patients' charts that were locked away and not available. Only the foreign, non-Vietnamese nurses worked on Sundays or holidays.[17]

It was extremely difficult for the U.S. nurses to train their counterparts in bedside care. The USAID advisors met with resistance to introducing even simple sterile techniques, and frequently the same dressing forceps was used for ten to twelve patients. Unfortunately, when the American nurse advisors attempted to teach sterile techniques, the Vietnamese nurses disappeared, and in essence, the more the American nurses did, the less the Vietnamese nurses were willing to learn or do for themselves.[18] The parallels between this aspect of providing health care and in how the war was fought are striking.

American nurses also feared that the training would not provide lasting benefits once the Americans left. As Medical Corps Maj. Glenn W. Dunnington (the officer in command of the 447th Medical Detachment Military Provincial Hospital Augmentation Program [MILPHAP] team in Pleiku and in charge of the training program) said, "I'm afraid that when I leave and the Vietnamese take over the surgical ward, the Vietnamese nurses will go back to their usual practices of not taking care of the patients."[19] This tendency of the Vietnamese to allow U.S. military and civilian advisors to carry out tasks rather than to learn to do them would persist throughout much of the war, both within the medical setting and elsewhere.

All health programs in South Vietnam suffered from a shortage of qualified personnel. This was due in part to the paltry health worker salaries, leading to significant flight of paramedical health workers into unrelated positions.[20] For example, nurses and trained technicians could earn more money working as interpreters for the Americans than remaining in the medical field. In my own experience, our battalion interpreter, Vi Hui, had been trained as a health care worker in the North before coming to the South. Dr. John H. Knowles, superintendent of Massachusetts General Hospital and part of a survey team of American physicians, noted that the South Vietnamese spent "less than 1 percent of their budget on health services, less than any other country, with or without a war" and that it was simply necessary to spend more money on health problems.[21]

Vietnam in the early to mid-1960s therefore represented a nation in conflict, where medical care to civilians had the potential to influence the outcome of that conflict. There was an inadequate health care system, both qualitatively and quantitatively. The war was fought for the allegiance of the rural population that was courted by both sides of the conflict. Medical care could partially determine which side would win the support of the people and win the war.

The first numerically significant U.S. forces in Vietnam were army SF. Their medical assistance program was not part of the formal MEDCAP to be described in the next chapter. The experiences of the SF were, in many ways, similar to those of the units participating in the later programs, although on a somewhat smaller scale.

The rural healers were respected figures within their communities. U.S. documents often referred to them as "witch doctors" or "sorcerers." An effort to win over and work with the local medicine man had been ignored in Vietnam early on, but the SF medics rapidly learned its benefit. Often they had great influence over the village chief. The SF medics worked with them so that they would not lose face; otherwise, they could prevent the medics from treating anyone in the village. "Sharing credit" was an effective technique to win over the village healers.[22]

The SF medical aid program emphasized using medical care to improve intelligence gathering more than the later MEDCAP I or II programs. As the SF units were located in the western parts of the country to a great extent, much of their effort was directed at providing medical care to the Civilian Irregular Defense Group (CIDG) units composed of Montagnards, Nuongs, and Cambodians. The Vietnamese and the GVN virtually despised these groups, to the extent that the GVN would not recognize or certify the non-Vietnamese trainees.[23] General Khanh considered the Montagnards to be enemies of the South Vietnamese, unreliable and liable to turn on the government.[24] They had previously unsuccessfully revolted against the government of South Vietnam. Many of these mountain tribesmen had never seen a doctor, about 35 percent had tuberculosis, close to 10 percent had leprosy (the highest rate in the world), and 75 percent of the children died in childbirth.[25]

More than 90 percent of the population of Vietnam lived on the coastal plain and in the Mekong Delta; the Central Highlands and the frontiers were essentially unpopulated. Eighty percent of the American forces came to be concentrated in areas containing less than 4 percent of the population to the extent that the locale of American military operations, largely against regular units of the North Vietnamese Army (NVA) (more properly, PAVN), was geographically removed from that of the guerilla conflict. As North Vietnamese writers have pointed out, the United States could not hold territory and protect the population at the same time.[26]

While the SF civic action was viewed by army headquarters as "wholly outside the formal Medical Civic Action Program,"[27] the SF considered the medics to be their "most valuable anti-guerilla asset."[28] On paper, SF supplies came through their own (SF) channels, with Okinawa a primary source of supply. In reality, this was time consuming and unreliable. Many medical supplies were obtained through the time-honored technique of "scrounging." In my own experience, I can testify to trading medical supplies to locally based SF units for war trophies such as souvenir captured weapons.

Each SF "A" team included two highly trained enlisted medical specialists capable of independent medical operation. These men provided medical care for their team members and the personnel they trained and organized into paramilitary forces and the civilians in their area of operations. The SF ability to improvise was exemplified by a June 1967 report regarding a patrol in the Cam-Lam sector. "A U.S. doctor, dentist, and veterinarian were there. Six hundred and fifty people were treated, plus one wounded water buffalo."[29] A difficulty with the program was that when the detachment was withdrawn or transferred, the medical programs effectively ceased.[30]

One SF medic told of how they would seek cases that would be easy to cure and obtain a dramatic result when they entered a village to impress the inhabitants. "If we see a kid running around with a case of ringworm, someone with a sty or a cyst or a swollen jaw, we practically kidnap him off the streets for treatment."[31] As maxillofacial surgeon Lt. Col. Richard Morgan put it, "In the case of cleft lip deformity, a single stage operation often changed a grotesque appearing child to one with a semblance of normalcy. The parents were ordinarily very grateful, and it helped the SF teams to gain some access with the local people."[32] Another dramatic example was a boy with congenital club feet, carried into the hospital by his mother and walking back into his village a month later.[33]

The SF A teams delivered most of the medical care to civilians in the early years of their involvement in Vietnam. Before 1965, the border surveillance sites in isolated areas did not offer the same opportunities for civic action that existed in the developed urban centers. Nevertheless, the SF, to the extent practical, ran medical dispensaries, helped build schools and local markets and initiated sanitation, agricultural, and home improvement projects in the isolated regions. The medics functioned virtually without any laboratory or radiology backup.

The SF ran the programs in a rather irregular manner. Charles Bartley, a SF medic, described "going out 10–20 Ks [kilometers] from camp. We did not work a particular system. You get involved in doing a daily routine, or weekly, and Charlie knows where you are."[34] Another SF medic, S.Sgt. David Tittsworth concurred, saying, "We would arbitrarily go there, maybe a few times a week." He added, the "purpose was of course a political one to show the local people that the government was concerned about their health and welfare."[35]

The teams emphasized sanitation procedures. SSG Scott Herbert, an SF medic, reported distributing large quantities of soap, which they trained the people to use. With medical supplies limited, "all we had was the soap." A "soap economy" developed, with the SF team paying with soap for work such as filling sandbags. The village began bartering and trading with soap, and "everyone was using soap."[36]

As the CIDG program developed, it became customary for the two medical noncommissioned officers in each A detachment to hold sick call at the CIDG dispensary or in the adjoining village. This occurred two or three times a week for the benefit of the CIDG dependents, the local villagers, and others from the surrounding countryside. Control of the supplies and medicines used in the CIDG facilities was tenuous. Barry Zindel, a Medical Corps officer serving with the SF, noted that many more medicines were given to the CIDG hospital than ever could have been used, and U.S. personnel were not allowed to inventory the pharmacy supplies. The hospital treated only minor problems, while they requisitioned "major type meds." S.Sgt. Herbert was reprimanded for refusing to give supplies to one of the Vietnamese medics after becoming suspicious about the large requests for medicines in the face of small sick call numbers. In an attempt to control losses, he insisted that all supplies be signed for by the CIDG medic, and he himself initialed each bottle of medicine as another control measure. The SF unit later caught a VC woman in the mountains with a full bottle of chloroquinine (an antimalarial drug) that he had initialed when it was issued to the dispensary.[37]

Efforts to provide a full therapeutic course of medication to the villagers were often problematic. People with no tradition of taking medicines over a period of time would tend to take all the pills at once, rather than a pill three times a day for two weeks. In addition, there was always the chance that the local VC would take the medicine away from the patient. One solution was to move the patient to a base camp where he could be given the medicines over the proper time span. This plan also created problems because when a Montagnard was evacuated, it was necessary to evacuate his entire family with him. If possible, the team would try to convince the patient to return on a daily basis for medicine. The medics also learned to observe the patients taking the medicine so that they would not spit out the pills and give them away later. At times, however, the patients would hold the medicine under their tongue until they could remove it later to give away.

Medic Bartley quickly learned the limitations of the program. "Initially I wanted to cure the whole damn country of all the diseases they had. I came to find out it is a little ridiculous to attempt. You treat on a day-to-day basis. You treat that particular disease."[38]

There was also a high incidence of venereal disease and cases of tuberculosis. The medics realized that some of the patients they treated were VC. As M.Sgt. James Whitener said, "It was too hard to distinguish who was who, so you treat the needy—and worry about whether they were VC or not later."[39] When in November 1965 Surgeon General Heaton visited Sadec, which was on the boundary of VC territory, he was told that at one time 90 percent of the patients seen by MEDCAP teams were VC, but "now there are only 10%."[40]

During a serious epidemic of gastroenteritis and typhoid fever at Moc Hoa in Kien Tuong Province, the refugee women and children treated were all said to be VC sympathizers.[41] The VC would also send in villagers with instructions as to which symptoms to describe to get medicine that the VC needed.[42] Training programs were also vulnerable to enemy infiltration. When discussing a training program for indigenous medics, Col. Valentine B. Sky told the interviewer, "On graduation day, two didn't show up, including the number one man in the class: they were both VC. They managed to sneak their people in to be trained how to use the American medicines."[43]

The noncommissioned officer medics of the SF also recognized that the medical civic action's purpose was primarily political. The program was designed to show the local people that the government was concerned about their health and welfare. Even treating the enemy was not necessarily a negative because it showed the population that the United States cared about them, regardless of politics. By doing so, the United States hoped to win VC sympathizers over to the side of the GVN. The contribution by the medics is "generally considered to be the most influential and productive of all the various civic action programs—and by far the biggest success with the people."[44] A significant question, which will be discussed in Chapters 6 and 7, is whether this activity by uniformed U.S. servicemen did, in fact, transfer over to the GVN or the goodwill accrued only to the U.S. forces.

Some of the experiences of the SF medics were perverse. James Whitener recounted a case where a man brought in his daughter, "a beautiful girl about 16 years old." She had broken her leg, and it had healed with a deformity causing her to walk on the bones of the leg with the ankle dragging. The medics wanted to arrange for her to go to a hospital to have the deformity corrected, which was clearly feasible. Her father refused to let her have it corrected, as she made her living begging and "no one would pay to see a normal girl walk around."[45] In another case, the medics had gained the trust of a villager who refused to let his wife deliver her baby until after the Americans saw her. He pushed the baby back inside his wife, resulting in the baby's death; the medics were able to save the mother.[46] In another instance, army medic

Sgt. Donald Wolford delivered healthy twins in a village near Plei Mrong. When he returned to check up on the family the next day, the mother had only one baby. They had thrown the other one away; it was bad luck to keep two.[47]

As noted earlier, medical services could also be useful in intelligence gathering. Medic Bartley noted that medical civic action was useful in establishing a rapport with the people. The servicemen learned about the health problems of the guerillas by the kinds of medicines they were trying to get from the villagers. On occasion, they would put a "tail" on a suspicious patient and watch and see him deliver the medicines to someone waiting out in the bush. Intelligence personnel from the Central Intelligence Agency (CIA) accompanied some MEDCAP missions. The CIA presence was sporadic, and they did not control the SF units. Sfc. Henry Shelly, working with the Montagnards, reported that the medics they were training in the villages received extra money for intelligence information.[48] Evidence of this occurred only in conjunction with the SF programs. Medical Corps LTC Gerald Foy, the 5th SF Group Surgeon, felt medical civic action was of little medical value but was useful as an intelligence cover.[49]

Much of this SF activity was very loosely controlled. To a great extent the activities were unsupervised; it was rare to have a physician present. Occasionally, a dentist would accompany the team, performing mainly extractive dentistry. Statistics were of dubious quality, as some units reported no medical statistics while others recorded seeing "maybe a couple of dozen people a day."[50]

The other organization that delivered medical care to the people outside of the formalized programs was the U.S. Marines in I Corps, the northern part of South Vietnam. The marines were the first large contingent of combat troops brought into the country in March 1965. They were initially assigned the task of protecting the air force base at Da Nang, but it rapidly became apparent that unless they were permitted to maneuver and patrol outside of the base camp, they would simply be sitting ducks in a defensive position. Ultimately, they were given primary responsibility for the U.S. operations in the northern-most corps tactical zone of the country, I Corps.

During the Korean conflict, marine ground and air forces had been under the operational control of the army and did not operate independently.[51] The marines hoped to avoid playing a support role to other services in Vietnam. With the marine forces (with the formal designation of III Marine Amphibious Force [III MAF]) carrying the main responsibility in I Corps and the army responsible for the remainder of the country, the marines were a primary force rather than in a supporting role. The senior Marine Corps officer was not only the commanding general, III MAF, but also the U.S. I Corps area coordinator and senior advisor. As Jack Shulimson notes, he was responsible for all U.S. forces in the five northern provinces that constituted I Corps.[52] Westmoreland, as head of MACV and USARV, exercised overall command in Vietnam. Marine administrative and logistical support came from the Fleet Marine Force Pacific, rather than from MACV and USARV. Marine strength in I Corps had risen to 81,000 by 1969.[53]

The army under Gen. William C. Westmoreland and the marines under Gen. Lewis W. Walt, supported by Lt. Gen. Victor H. Krulak Jr. at Fleet Marine Force Pacific, differed as to the best way to fight the war.[54] Walt was under the operational control of MACV, but greatly influenced by Krulak's strong personality and experience, rather than as a function of the direct operational chain of command. Westmoreland and his staff focused on the defeat of the enemy main force. Accordingly, his primary goal was to track down the Communist main force units in the bush and bring them to battle.[55] This was in spite of the fact that well over 80 percent of significant contacts with the enemy were initiated by the enemy, at times and places of their choosing and often with an ability to break off contact and fade into the jungle if they saw fit to do so. This enabled the enemy to basically control the level of their casualties.

Westmoreland thought the marines were too "infatuated"

with holding real estate and in civic action were too widely dispersed and too hesitant to conduct offensive maneuvers. In an army Chief of Staff meeting, Lt. Gen. John Throckmorton (deputy commander of MACV) noted that when the marines were first deployed to Vietnam, they steadfastly refused to participate in search and destroy missions. Westmoreland, Throckmorton said, believed that the Marine concept of operations was wrong.[56] The commandant of the Marine Corps, Gen. Wallace M. Greene Jr., maintained that only a deliberate and necessarily slow expansion of the enclaves could provide rural security. With the villagers on their side, the marines believed they could break the connection between the guerrillas and the infrastructure within the enemy main force.[57] In part, this dispute arose from the convoluted command structure in Vietnam to which I have previously alluded. Westmoreland was unable to simply impose his will on the marines to have a uniform approach to fighting the war throughout the country.

Jim Seaton described these different schools of thought as a dominant school aiming to crush the enemy with an iron fist of military might and the lesser one seeking to strain the guerilla out of the population. This metaphor meshes nicely with Mao Tse Tung's concept regarding guerilla warfare—the "people are like the water and the army is like the fish."[58] The army's insistence on aggressive military operations pushed the pacification campaign seeking the VC cadres in the hamlets into secondary status, in other words, what the Communists put first (the villages and hamlets), the U.S. Army put second (after seeking the main force units).[59]

The Marine Corps leaders argued that small unit operations designed to protect the people against the guerrillas, combined with action against larger enemy forces when possible in conditions favorable to U.S. forces was the correct way to conduct the war. But the marines never made any headway with Westmoreland with this argument. Attempts to persuade McNamara and then to present the concept to President Johnson came to naught. In their discussions of the Combined Action Platoon (CAP) program, both Blaufarb of the CIA and political scientist Krepinevich felt it could have been effective and produced lower casualty rates than Westmoreland's tactics.[60]

While the marines felt strongly regarding the differences in their approach to pacification, neither they nor Westmoreland wanted the issue to come to a head. As Shulimson put it, "Rather than directly challenge the authority of the marine commanders, General Westmoreland preferred to issue orders for specific projects," which would get the marines to conduct the war more as he wished.[61] Even so, the marine leaders publicly defended their program. They felt that large unit ground actions were ultimately effective only if they reinforced the stability of the GVN and advanced its survival plan. As late as 1971, Secretary of the Navy John Chafee could state that no hamlet or village with a CAP presence had reverted to VC control.[62] Some of the wartime critics of the program later praised it and its limited success, even implying that they had supported it wholeheartedly throughout the conflict.[63]

When in 1967 the Civil Operations, Revolutionary Development Support (CORDS) organization took over responsibility for support of the pacification program, it superseded the marine effort in I Corps. This occurred simultaneously with a greater emphasis on a more traditional combat role for the marines, opposing the increased NVA incursions across the DMZ and through northern Laos.

These programs, one conducted by the army SF units and the other by the Marine Corps, treated many Vietnamese civilians in the villages and hamlets. The care was rendered by enlisted corpsmen, with only occasional visits from doctors, dentists, nurses, or veterinarians. The level of medical care they provided was even more rudimentary than that generally seen within the more formalized MEDCAP programs. Neither of these groups kept medical records on the patients, and the numbers of those treated can only be considered as approximations. They established long-term relationships with their villages and hamlets and with the local irregular defense forces.

The prolonged presence of the units within the villages and hamlets created a feeling of camaraderie and unity with the Vietnamese people. As the people came to trust the Americans and believe they would stay for a long time, they provided information regarding enemy activities and whereabouts. This, in turn, enabled the American units to provide better security for the villagers. Hamlets and villages thus moved from disputed control to the side of the GVN.

While the military and humanitarian efforts were conducted primarily by the United States, other countries also offered their support. The U.S. government (and especially President Johnson) deeply desired that other "free world" nations take part in the effort and it not be solely an American conflict. Medical teams also came to Vietnam from Korea, Nationalist China, Australia, New Zealand, Britain, Canada, Spain, Iran, the Philippines, and Switzerland.[64] The West German hospital ship *Heligoland* reached Saigon on 14 September 1966.[65] Japan and Italy also sent hospital ships.

The Philippines had a contingent of civilian doctors and nurses in Vietnam since before the Geneva agreement of 1954. This privately sponsored group arrived in 1953. The year after the Geneva accords, 1955, the group acquired official government status and was named the Philippine Contingent to Vietnam (Philcon V).[66]

In the middle of 1966, in response to the Republic of Vietnam request for additional assistance, the Philippine government augmented the Philcon V with the Philippine Civic Action Group, Vietnam (PHILCAGV), adding engineering works to the basic mission. PHILCAGV was activated 9 June 1966, when the Philippine Congress authorized the government to send a contingent to

Vietnam composed of engineer/construction, medical, and rural development personnel. The legislation also provided for an allocation of funds up to 35 million pesos ($8,950,000). The mission of the Philippine group was "to render civic action assistance to the Republic of Vietnam by construction, rehabilitation, and development of public works, utilities and structures, and by providing technical advice on other socio-economic activities." The medical unit set up a clinic equipped to perform minor surgery and provide dental care.

The Philippine contingent's constant reiteration of their nonaggressive and constructive mission, the fact that they were Asian, which deflected the anticolonial anti-European attitudes of the Vietnamese people, and the frequent ability of their medical teams to deal with the Vietnamese in their own language engendered very positive attitudes toward PHILCAGV by the people. Medical-surgical teams worked in Tay Ninh, Binh Duong, and Dinh Tuong Province Hospitals, and a fourth rural health team worked in Hau Nghia Province.[67] The tour of duty for the Philippine team personnel was one year, paralleling that of U.S. personnel.

USAID also contracted with the International Rescue Committee to render aid to the civilian population of Vietnam. Fifty percent of the personnel serving under that contract were Cuban refugees. British, Canadian, Spanish, Dutch, Venezuelan, Haitian, and Greek personnel were also employed. The government of Canada supplied vaccines, supported a Canadian tuberculosis specialty team, and provided ten civilian defense hospital units, including two thousand hospital beds.[68]

During this period before the major U.S. military buildup of troops in Vietnam, medical aid to civilians can be characterized as being loosely organized, mainly in small units, and without the major command emphasis that would be seen at a later time. The motivation in many instances was altruism and humanitarianism. It also served to establish a rapport with the people. While

U.S. military commanders hoped to keep the doctors busy, there was not the formal requirement for medical civic action programs that would accompany the arrival of large units into the country. More often than not, participation in the care of civilians, refugees, and orphans was undertaken by medical sections due to their own desire to keep busy. The SF especially gathered some intelligence in the hinterlands, but it was casual, sporadic, and very local in nature. The monetary expenditures involved in the programs were not large. The system had yet to be formalized.

The proliferation of organizations that were quasimilitary, quasicivilian, or some mixture of the two created a plethora of alphabet soup and confusion. There were organizations that were U.S. military, U.S. military in conjunction with Vietnamese counterparts, or U.S. military in combination with Vietnamese civilian organizations. There were no clear lines of responsibility or command. Funding was obtained from multiple sources, controlled by the Vietnamese Ministry of Health (MOH), the Vietnamese military, the U.S. military, and the U.S. State Department through USAID (with some CIA input). Programs overlapped in responsibility and geography. Lines of demarcation were unclear. There was a need for some controlling organization able to work with both civilians and the military, as well as both the Free World Military Assistance Forces (FWMAF) and the Vietnamese. Enter CORDS.

In an initial attempt to coordinate all U.S. civilian pacification programs, Deputy Ambassador William Porter established the Office of Civil Operations (OCO) in December 1966. It placed all U.S. civilian advisory efforts under a single representative at the provincial and military regional levels. OCO never really took hold, as cooperation and coordination was voluntary by operatives of USAID, Office of the Special Assistant (OSA), and Joint U.S. Public Affairs Office (JUSPAO), which combined U.S. Information Service (USIS) and psychological operations elements. Each of these agencies was autonomous and dealt directly with its own Washington headquarters.[69]

The military did not think that OCO would succeed and prepared for that eventuality. Gen. Harold K. Johnson, army chief of staff, foresaw "a major problem of interface between MACV staff and OCO."[70] Wheeler directed Westmoreland to establish a channel between the embassy and his headquarters and prepare to transfer the authority and direction of the pacification operation into MACV.[71] Col. (later Maj. Gen.) Harris Hollis (who was placed in Porter's office while retaining his position as the MACV J-3) fulfilled that role. Westmoreland also realized that the civilian effort in the embassy was bound to fail and created the MACV Revolutionary Development Support Directorate headed by Brig. Gen. William Knowlton. Westmoreland later said, "Porter had an impossible job to do in Vietnam and wasn't staffed to do it. As a result, MACV took over the Civil Operations, Revolutionary Support Development organization" (for the directive establishing CORDS, see Appendix B).[72]

President Johnson signed the National Security Action Memo creating CORDS on 9 May 1967.[73] This move required the integration of approximately twelve hundred civilians under MACV.[74] Robert W. Komer was named deputy to the commander of MACV for pacification with the personal rank of ambassador.[75] Historian Thomas W. Scoville gives three "compelling reasons" for the changes. First, normal governmental coordination was inadequate for the interwoven civil and military agencies involved with pacification. Second, the pacification problem was simply too large and complex for the civilian agencies to handle alone. Third, pacification was failing in part because of lack of security, and the military would take the need for security more seriously if it was responsible for pacification.[76]

Komer considered that the programs differed from their predecessors less in concept than in the comprehensive nature and massive scale of the effort and the unified management system. He also realized the difficulty in evaluating the programs: "Even over the short-term, however, it is hard to assess the *relative* extent to which undoubted changes in the countryside can be properly attributed to the *pacification* program as opposed to other factors" [emphasis in the original]. And, "in an unconventional conflict like Vietnam the relative impact of pacification versus other political, military, or psychological factors is exceedingly hard to sort out."[77]

Not even Komer could gain control over all the civilian agencies. Brig. Gen. Philip Bolté recalled that when he served as an advisor in Quang Tin Province in I Corps, he thought he was in charge of all the pacification programs operating in the area. He soon found that this did not include CIA operations, over which he had no control.[78] Rick Kiernan, who served on an advisory team in Hau Nghia Province as an army major, described CORDS as "a kind of small government," with teams of specialists from the State Department, Department of Defense, CIA, and the Department of Agriculture.[79]

Komer believed that pacification was as much a military as a civilian process, because there could be no civil progress without constant real security. Most of the security forces needed were under the U.S. and ARVN military, and without them, pacification in the countryside could not be expanded rapidly enough to exploit success in pushing back the enemy main forces. Further, Komer pointed out that the military are "far better able to organize, manage and execute major field problems under chaotic wartime conditions than are civilian agencies."[80]

CORDS has been described as a "matrix organization."[81] Matrix organizations are those in which specialists are drawn from functional departments or organizations to work on projects, either one time or ongoing. The specialists remain assigned to their parent organizations but give operational efforts to the project director. Authority over such project people thus come from two directions, with the crossing lines of authority viewed as a "matrix." This created an unusual situation in which civilians were in charge of military personnel in an active war, and it was especially significant for the career officer whose evaluations

(Officer Efficiency Reports [OERs]) were critical to promotion and a long-term career. One result of this was that in spite of many efforts to rectify this problem, many top-quality officers felt their careers would be adversely affected by serving as advisors rather than in combat command positions and refused those assignments.

As an organization melding soldiers and civilians, CORDS had no real precedent. The overwhelming presence was that of the military component. One CORDS official likened it to "an elephant and rabbit stew—one elephant and one rabbit."[82] Formed at the behest of President Johnson, it ended in January 1973 when the Paris Accords went into effect. An entirely civilian operation headed by George Jacobson (special assistant to the ambassador) assumed its functions and programs. Jacobson had previously served in CORDS.[83]

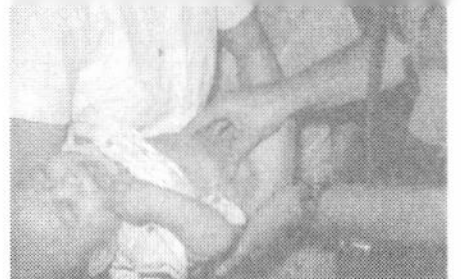

Four

Formal MEDCAP, CAP, MILPHAP, and CWCP

The military loves acronyms. Every major program or title becomes known by its initials or abbreviations, most pronounceable as a word or phrase. The various military medical programs are no exception. Their use provides convenient shorthand in both writing and speaking and minimizes lengthy repetitions. Further, these words take on their own life. The Medical Civic Action Program became MEDCAP. When the program was modified, the old one, MEDCAP, became MEDCAP I and the new one MEDCAP II. Other programs utilizing acronyms under consideration were the Military Provincial Hospital Augmentation Program, later changed to the Military Provincial Health Program, but both used the acronym of MILPHAP, the Civilian War Casualty Program (CWCP), the Provincial Health Assistance Program (PHAP), and the previously discussed Marine Combined Action Platoons (CAP).

In September 1961, Congress created the Agency for International Development (AID), sometimes referred to as the USAID. During the 1960s, AID funneled $47 billion to development programs worldwide.[1] The formation of AID shifted the responsibility for administering the development of health care delivery systems in lesser-developed countries to the State Department.[2] AID could contract with nonprofit agencies such as church groups or Project Health Opportunities for People Everywhere (Project HOPE) to implement its programs. If the administration of the programs occurred through nongovernmental organizations (NGOs), the recipients of the benefits might not even realize that their benefactor was the U.S. government.[3]

Civilian NGOs were active in Vietnam in the 1950s and 1960s. The *S.S. Hope,* the ship of Project HOPE, visited Saigon with a volunteer physician staff and personnel. They considered local customs of midwifery and witch doctors to be deterrents to good health and found a "pathetic" prevalence of polio among children.[4] A program called Orthopedics Overseas began in November 1961.[5] By December 1964, more than sixty American physicians had paid their own way to Vietnam, most for very short periods of thirty to sixty days. There they trained Vietnamese physicians while caring for the sick and injured.

While the medical programs in Vietnam began under the Department of State and various volunteer organizations, such as Project HOPE, Cooperative for American Relief Everywhere (CARE), and religious groups, the military ultimately dominated and controlled them. Unlike the volunteer programs that lacked political intentions, the medical programs operating under various governmental agencies served at least two purposes. First, medical training, education, and support programs helped (or at least hoped) to make the Vietnamese capable of maintaining a satisfactory level of preventive and therapeutic medicine. Second, the programs sought to enhance the overall prestige of the government of Vietnam and win the hearts and minds of the Vietnamese people.[6] These programs began during the period of the MAAG, when the U.S. military presence was small and mainly in an advisory role. The financial outlay for them was minimal.

Initially, the United States intended to have physicians from nations friendly to Vietnam volunteer for a tour of duty there to replace civilian Vietnamese physicians who would then treat people in the remote villages. This idea was dropped when it became apparent that Vietnamese physicians did not want their practices in the hands of foreigners. In any case, there was an inadequate number of Vietnamese physicians available to implement this program. Next, the United States considered recruiting physicians from the United States and commissioning them in the USPHS. Yet again, there were not enough volunteers to make this idea worthwhile.

There was a short-lived Volunteer Physicians for Vietnam Program. It was conducted in coordination with the American Medical Association, and volunteer physicians went to Vietnam for sixty-, ninety-, or 120-day tours. While the caliber of the physicians was high, it could not be sustained. The adventure became less attractive as the war increased in intensity. The number of volunteers was inadequate, creating vacancies. The tours were too short to enable the physicians to develop a significant relationship with their Vietnamese counterparts. While good work was unquestionably done, it was of limited impact on the situation in the country.

Dr. Patricia Smith had worked in the Central Highlands with the Montagnards since July 1959. Kontum had the highest leprosy rate in the world, and 40 percent of the people had tuberculosis.[7] The Montagnard language has no word for doctor; the tribesmen called Dr. Smith *Ya Pogang*, Honorable Lady of Medicine. She went to Vietnam under the auspices of Catholic Relief Services, an agency of the National Catholic Welfare Conference. Initially there was a dispensary, which was expanded into a hospital in May 1963. She remained there until the end of U.S. involvement in Vietnam. No attempt was made to ascertain the political leanings of her patients; all were treated as needed. Most certainly some were VC.

Even before the major U.S. troop buildup, the administration recognized the need for rural medical care in Vietnam. The State Department sent a telegram indicating this to the MAAG in April

1962.[8] In his report to Gen. Paul D. Harkins, (Commander, USMACV), in October 1962, Australian Col. F. P. Serong[9] noted deterioration in the Vietnamese village medic program, which he considered "the keystone of our civic action work—and of our intelligence net."[10] The village medics were abandoning their posts because they were not being paid. He further noted the "inherent danger" in allowing a military project to be supported in vital areas by a "civilian project over which the military has no control." Finally, the U.S. Army took charge of the responsibility of furnishing physicians and enlisted medical technicians. The MAAG personnel roles were revised to accept this additional responsibility.

PHAP/AGHD

PHAP embodied most of the field operating elements and resources of USAID's program of public health assistance to the GVN Ministry of Health, Social Welfare and Refugees (MHSWR). Thus it was a State Department program operating under the supervision of USAID personnel and was, therefore, not primarily a military program.[11] It was a multinational assistance effort to give direct medical and health care to Vietnamese and expand Vietnamese capabilities in clinical health care.[12] As one of the main objectives of the program was to augment and strengthen the Vietnamese medical capabilities, it was important that Vietnamese rather than U.S. or free-world forces render the care. PHAP aimed to achieve an immediate increase in the capabilities of GVN Provincial and Prefectural Health Services through temporary augmentation by U.S. and Free World Assistance personnel and materials and foster permanent improvement in these health services through advice and assistance. The first team of U.S. civilian physicians, nurses, and technicians arrived in Can Tho in the summer of 1962. It aimed to improve the training of their Vietnamese counterparts, that is the physicians, nurses, and technicians.[13]

PHAP was designed to be of short-term duration, being phased out of existence as soon as feasible. In each province a USAID medical officer in charge was designated who worked under the Vietnamese Chief Health Officer (CHO) of the regional entity. According to regulation, it was the responsibility of military medical advisors serving in command staff positions to coordinate civilian medical programs with the GVN province medical chief and the medical officer of PHAP.[14] To an extent, the significance of PHAP is that it was another example of the military/civilian aid interface.

It also was another example of the difficulty in coordinating the various programs with the GVN. A special organization within the Vietnamese MOH was created in 1964 to manage the health development project supported by USAID. It was called the Administration General for Health Development (AGHD) with the primary purpose to direct and supervise all activities supported by USAID in Vietnam. The AGHD was never accepted by the main body of the MOH, mainly because of internal organizational fighting over control of funds and other resources. The organization was conceived as a means of bypassing the regular establishment of the MOH and cutting through the bureaucracy. A general attitude prevailed within the MOH that the AGHD was "USAID's baby" and not really a part of the Health Ministry.[15] This example of bureaucratic infighting was to be repeated on multiple occasions throughout the war.

The AGHD struggled in its early organizational phase, was never seen as a partner by the MOH, and never established a firm political base. The MOH viewed it as a competitor for resources and power. The AGHD also had difficulties with the Director General of the Budget and Foreign Aid of the GVN. By the summer of 1965, the AGHD had lost steam, and with the exception of the flow of a few commodities and the ongoing construction at several provincial hospitals, was accomplishing little.

Air Force Maj. Gen. James W. Humphreys Jr., a Medical Corps officer, was loaned to USAID as assistant director for public health. It was envisioned that the majority of the effort should be placed on the rural health development and public health practices. In General Humphreys' view, the efforts of both USAID and the MOH were divided and inefficient. The immunization program was "spotty" and not receiving good support from the Vietnamese side in spite of pressure from USAID. Public health nurses in the field were moved from province to province, diluting their efforts. The malaria eradication program suffered from inability to get at those areas with the highest levels of endemic disease because of inadequate security and loss of malaria advisors. Hospital facilities dated from the late 1800s and early 1900s; 90 percent were without running water and had little or no power and no sewage disposal systems. Equipment was old and a mixture of old French and modern donations from many countries, with no maintenance capability.[16] More than six thousand hamlets required health stations.

MEDCAP and CAP

In November 1962, approval was obtained to initiate a MEDCAP in the Republic of Vietnam. It was implemented two months later on 27 January 1963.[17] From its inception, MEDCAP was to be primarily a political and psychological tool.[18] It was initiated as part of a countrywide civic action program. The basic intent of MEDCAP was to "establish and maintain a continuing spirit of mutual respect and cooperation between the Republic of Vietnam Armed Forces (RVNAF) and the civilian population."[19] Note the two sides mentioned, the RVNAF and the people, not the U.S. armed forces and the people. The program's objectives were to convince the people in the remote areas that the government was vitally interested in their welfare, encourage the Vietnamese public health agencies to cooperate with and include civic action in their rural health endeavors, and provide instruction to village health workers.

The first American MEDCAP teams arrived in Vietnam in January 1963. They arrived without adequate orientation on the environment, language, culture, and medical problems they would have to face. U.S. medical personnel were assigned to assist the Vietnamese medical personnel, and a "bonus" side effect was the improvement of the image of the U.S. medical personnel. From the start, the province chiefs' cooperation with MEDCAP teams varied from excellent to unsatisfactory levels. Supplies for the program were funded by U.S. Overseas Mission (USOM) and distributed through existing Vietnamese medical depots. In 1964, the cost of supplies expended totaled $583,091.[20]

Initially, the Department of the Army furnished personnel for MEDCAP teams. In January 1963, the 127 members were divided into twenty-nine teams and assigned to nine ARVN divisions, separate regiments, Regional Forces and Popular Forces (RF/PF) units, and each corps. The initial group of physicians and enlisted medical personnel were sent to Vietnam on temporary duty orders (TDY) from Okinawa and Japan for a period not to exceed 150 days.[21] This occurred before the insertion of U.S. combat forces in March 1965.

In December 1963, fifty-four medical spaces were eliminated from the program as a first step in the U.S. phase-out, intended to be completed by June 1964. The phase-out was based on the assumption that Vietnamese Army MEDCAP teams were capable of assuming the full responsibility for the program.[22] The COMUSMACV approved the continuation of the U.S. participation through the end of 1964 because the MAAG surgeon, Col. Thomas A. Britton, felt the Vietnamese teams were not ready to assume full responsibility. As of 1 January 1965, MEDCAP became a program carried on by Vietnamese medical personnel, with U.S. medical personnel acting in an advisory capacity. In mid-1966, 86 percent of the total teams operating in Vietnam were Vietnamese.[23] Finally, in June 1967, this program (renamed as MEDCAP I) officially became the full responsibility of the ARVN.[24] Thus, the original MEDCAP program of American teams aiding Vietnamese medical personnel was converted into a program run by the Vietnamese Army. Yet neither of these concepts are what most think of when the term MEDCAP is used.

The original program was meant to improve the image of the Vietnamese Army in the eyes of the civilian population. It had the potential to transcend distrust or even dislike of the central government on the part of the general population. This was to be accomplished through the use of Vietnamese military and paramilitary forces. It was recognized early on that U.S. medical personnel in uniform rendering the treatments could not achieve an improvement in the image of the South Vietnamese Army.[25]

The introduction of large bodies of American troops into Vietnam in 1965 meant that many American medical personnel became available to provide care for the Vietnamese. Military units of the United States and FWMAF assumed responsibility for civilians within their areas of operation, using the medical personnel assigned to their units. MEDCAP was the personification of Americans' view of their soldiers and the military helping civilians. U.S. Army surgeon, Maj. Gen. Spurgeon Neel, referred to it as the best known of the various medical civilian assistance programs.[26]

This program became known as MEDCAP II, with the original program, now run by the Vietnamese Army, renamed MEDCAP I. There was no longer any program officially known as simply MEDCAP. As with many other military acronyms, the term could be used as a verb, as in to MEDCAP, a noun, as in going on a MEDCAP, or an adjective, as in MEDCAP supplies.

In his 1965 message to Congress, President Johnson requested seven million dollars to provide improved medical and surgical services, "especially in the more remote areas of Vietnam, Laos, and Thailand." He noted that members of the American Medical Association had agreed to help recruit fifty surgeons and specialists to go to Vietnam to "help heal the wounds of war as well as the ravages of unchecked disease."[27] The president said he "was contemplating the expansion of existing programs under which mobile medical teams travel throughout the countryside providing on-the-spot medical facilities, treatment, and training in rural areas."[28] In early May 1965, Maj. Gen. Conn L. Milburn Jr., deputy surgeon general of the army, was sent to Vietnam to assist in formulating an expanded program of medical assistance to the people.

A medical policy coordinating committee was established in 1965 to plan and coordinate the growing number of medical programs involving aid to Vietnamese civilians. Headed jointly by the assistant director for public health (AID) and the MACV surgeon, the committee also included the surgeons of the MACV component commands.

It was not until President Johnson put the full weight of the U.S. government behind civic action in 1966 that the program gained momentum.[29] Duplications in services and programs under military auspices and under the State Department created inefficiencies that were heightened by interservice (army, navy, marines, and air force) and interdepartmental rivalries. Conflicts between the Saigon embassy and the Joint Chiefs of Staff in the Pentagon, as well as organizations such as USAID, U.S. Information Agency (USIA), and the CIA for control of the war were also reflected in jurisdictional battles in the pacification arena.[30]

Coordination of the various programs proved difficult throughout the conflict. On more than one occasion, a medical group under the auspices of one organization would arrive in a hamlet or orphanage to find another medical group working for a different organization already there or having just been there.[31] Artillery Col. Alfred Kitts commented that, at times, it seemed there were three separate campaigns in Binh Duong: the U.S. military effort, the ARVN effort, and the province pacification program. A "ridiculous" example of this happened in one hamlet when five separate U.S. civic action events occurred simultaneously. A U.S. artillery unit had arranged to sponsor the hamlet, but another division had two brigade MEDCAPs in progress, a U.S. hospital unit was conducting a DENTCAP, and the U.S. Navy was also offering medical care. None of the five agencies had coordinated their plans with district or province advisors for "security reasons."[32] While medical programs were only one facet of the pacification effort, they were a significant one.

Unlike MEDCAP I, MEDCAP II did not rely on a Vietnamese counterpart. It was under the auspices of MACV rather than MAAG and was, in part, a function of a much larger body of personnel to utilize. This resulted in virtually countrywide coverage, rather than the limited number of teams of the original program. MEDCAP II entailed the direct delivery of medical care to Vietnamese civilians by uniformed U.S. military medical personnel. This implied a difference in mission, as clearly its aim was not to build up support for the ARVN. It was more formalized than the *ad hoc* programs run by the SF units in regard to written plans and concurrence of the GVN, the USOM provincial representative, and the MACV sector advisor. MACV mandated monthly reports from each unit.[33] MEDCAP II acted in areas where civilian medical resources did not exist and did not compete with civilian practitioners. Competition with civilian medical activities was specifically prohibited by the regulation.[34] This competition with civilian care had been a problem under the previous more loosely organized programs. As Medical Corps Maj. John Reed of the 5th SF Group recalls, "We often got complaints that we were interfering with the livelihood of the Vietnamese physicians."[35]

The purpose of MEDCAP II was to win the confidence and gain the cooperation of the local population in areas where relatively large U.S. military forces were stationed. The delivery of care especially focused on children—giving vaccinations and cleaning up skin problems, providing food and clothing, and taking care of orphanages. This is why there were so many photographs of happy children by the roadside waving at the passing American soldiers. There was a problem with medications, however, as most army medicines were for adults, rather than in doses or preparations for children.[36]

Unit MEDCAP reports only provided a generalized overview of activities and often generalized in regard to treatments or numbers of patients seen. For example, the 52nd Artillery Group Army Medical Service Activities Report dated 26 January 1967 reported: "*Medical Civic Action*: A formal MEDCAP II Plan was submitted in accordance with USARV Reg 40–39 and was approved in November 1966. This program provides for regular MEDCAP visits to four villages near the base camp and to other hamlets which vary according to the changing locations of our firing batteries."

In the section of the report labeled "Civilian Activities," the MEDCAP is described as follows: "One of the most rewarding programs has been liaison activities with the indigenous population, the MEDCAP program. Periodic visits to both Montagnard and Vietnamese villages have proven beneficial to all concerned. In those villages which are visited regularly, iron and vitamins are dispensed to curb the nutritional deficiencies in the population. Most of the illnesses encountered have responded to minimal amount of care; soap and water with instructions in cleanliness have been the most effective therapy. An average of four hundred civilians each month are seen."[37]

There is a danger in drawing conclusions based on such estimates. One can easily imagine a clerk at the headquarters receiving this report and filling in the box on the consolidated report with 4,800 persons treated for the year (12 times 400 = 4,800), and from that moment on, an estimated figure becomes a hard statistic.

The army medical service activities reports frequently drew conclusions from generalized estimations without verifying data or explaining how the evaluations were made. In the 1st Battalion, 8th Artillery "approximately" three MedCAPs [*sic*] are carried out each month, treating an average of twenty-five civilians per MEDCAP.[38] The 2nd Battalion, 14th Infantry, 25th Division reported conducting "MEDCAPs five to six times per week treating eighty to one hundred Vietnamese on each day." The report concludes that "through the treatment performed on the Vietnamese, a larger number of the people have begun to better understand the American soldier and his presence in Vietnam. The Vietnamese people have accepted the program with great enthusiasm."[39] This implies a greater contact and exchange of thoughts and ideas than can be demonstrated. Many such impressions, both positive and negative, are contained in these reports without any evidence to support them and, as such, are of questionable reliability.

There were problems in instituting a MEDCAP program. The time required for beginning a program varied from six to twelve weeks. Approximately half of this time occurred while awaiting approval by various GVN, USOM, and MACV officials. This delay recurred whenever the unit moved to a new location (not exactly unusual in a war zone) or there was a change in the unit command or Medical Corps officer (the doctor). Twelve weeks constituted one-quarter of the one-year tour. Continuity in the programs remained a problem throughout the U.S. involvement in Vietnam.

All MEDCAP II projects needed the submission of a formal MEDCAP II plan approved by the MACV commander. The plan needed to include (1) areas to be covered pertaining to location and, where applicable, the specific type of project (e.g., leprosariums, orphanages, and refugee camps), (2) written approval of the Provincial Committee, and (3) provisions for coordination with the province medical chief. Only upon receiving approval for a plan could supply authorization and an account number be issued to requisition expendable medical supplies. The time from initial requisition to first issue of supplies was usually in excess of three weeks.[40] To counter these problems, many MEDCAP type missions were carried out unofficially, utilizing the supplies on hand

rather than those specifically intended for civic action (this was true in my personal experience on numerous occasions). This, of course, distorted the financial accounting for the program in that supplies for MEDCAP and unit support came from different sources and accounts. It contributes to the difficulty in accurately determining how much money was spent on the program.

To obtain the related goals of establishing mutual respect and cooperation and supporting Revolutionary Development, MACV established three objectives: (1) continuity, (2) participation, and (3) improvement of the health of the community.[41] First, to achieve continuity, MEDCAP must have a level of commitment that permitted scheduled participation and at a level of sophistication that local GVN health resources could sustain upon withdrawal of the U.S. military units. Second, local government representatives must participate in MEDCAP projects to train local Vietnamese health workers. Thus, MEDCAP intended to improve existing local health. Even so, sophisticated medical care and treatment was introduced only to the extent that facilities and equipment could be maintained by the GVN following ultimate U.S. withdrawal.

U.S. and FWMAF troop units of battalion size or larger conducted MEDCAP II. Despite the formal differences with the SF and marine CAP programs, there were great tactical similarities. Most of the cases seen were dermatological problems, mainly because of hygiene. Soap became a major instrument of care.[42] All FWMAF commanders were encouraged to have their forces participate in the program. While enhancing the prestige of the GVN remained desirous, the major U.S. military units had medical components with increased and underutilized capabilities. It was not thought possible to accomplish the program aims only through Vietnamese personnel.[43]

Commanders frequently referred to MEDCAP activities as voluntary. Personal experience by the author contradicts that concept. In a war where progress was measured by numbers, either of enemy killed or civilians immunized, unit commanders down to the battalion level had a vested interest in subtly and not so subtly encouraging their medical personnel to participate in the program. In a wonderfully worded example of military-speak, Medical Corps Col. Charles Mitchell describes the participation as "an added duty to be done in off-duty time."[44] This, of course, ignores the fact that almost all MEDCAPs were carried out during normal daylight duty hours and that the concept of off-duty time in a war zone is slightly ludicrous. Brig. Gen. James A. Wier, the USARV surgeon, recalls the unheeded objections by medical corps officers regarding participation in the program. Once the unit commander had volunteered the unit, the officers had to participate.[45]

The marine CAP was perhaps more closely analogous to the army SF programs than to any other program. In this case, CAP did not mean Civic Action Program, an error that appears frequently. Marines had used similar programs in the past, in Haiti (1915–34), Nicaragua (1926–33), and Santo Domingo (1916–22).[46] Capt. John J. Mullen Jr., 3rd Battalion, 4th Marines civil affairs officer, proposed the use of the program to make up for the scarcity of combat troops available to cover their Tactical Area of Operational Responsibility (TAOR).[47]

The CAP began in 1965 in Da Nang under marine Maj. Gen. (later Gen.) Lewis W. Walt, commander of the III MAF. His superior, Lt. Gen. Victor H. "Brute" Krulak, Commanding General, Fleet Marine Force, Pacific, also gave the program his "wholehearted support."[48] Like much of the American involvement in Vietnam, the program evolved extemporaneously.[49] At its peak, there were 114 combined action platoons throughout I Corps. According to Department of Defense (DOD), from 1 November 1967 through 31 January 1968, 49 percent of enemy initiated activity in I Corps occurred against CAPs. The CAPs quickly became primary targets for VC attacks.[50] This indicated both their position of vulnerability in the hamlets, as well as their desirability as a target worth attacking.

The first mission of each CAP was to provide security for the 

rural Vietnamese. The objectives of the Combined Action Force dictated that the area was essentially under VC influence and, therefore, hostile. The marines quickly realized that winning the support of the people was just as important as winning the battle against the VC. The people were neither friendly, nor unfriendly; they were seeking only survival.

Each combined action platoon was composed of fourteen U.S. Marines in a reinforced rifle squad (reinforced by a grenadier), one U.S. Naval hospital corpsman, and thirty-five Popular Force (PF) Vietnamese (a paramilitary force from the hamlets). Naval corpsmen and physicians were assigned to Marine forces to provide medical support. There was no separation between the U.S. and Vietnamese forces. They shared rations and quarters, and trained and fought side by side. Each CAP was assigned to a nearby U.S. Marine Corps infantry battalion for operational control that provided fire support as required.[51] Team members were volunteers, and at least one of them spoke Vietnamese.[52]

The CAP could not accomplish its objective of destroying the VC infrastructure without first being able to identify them. For this reason, they participated in civic action and psychological operations (psyops), and they were completely mobile within their TAOR. Success was achieved by building a bond between marine rifle squads and the population through a long-term presence. They stayed in their assigned hamlet twenty-four hours a day and did not go back to a U.S. base camp.

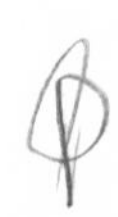

The corpsman was an indispensable link between the CAP and the civilians. His medical treatment was of a superficial nature, basically first aid and hygiene. Frequently, children were the first to visit, hopefully followed by the older members of the community. Hospital Corpsman 2nd Class Jerome McCart found that during his first tour in Vietnam, the team had "to seek out people needing medical aid when we entered a village," but on his second tour, the people came to seek out the team for treatment.[53] This occurred in combination with the team's interdiction of the

VC. This created movement of the "fence sitters" to the GVN-U.S. side. Ultimately, the population began to provide intelligence to the CAP that made the tactical operations more successful. Lieutenant General Walt cited instances of children warning the marines of booby traps, women showing where VC rice was stored, and others informing when the VC would come to collect taxes.[54]

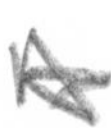

Every CAP corpsman had the added responsibility of training his Vietnamese PF counterpart. The district chief designated the PF corpsman who was most likely uneducated, ill trained, and ill equipped. The navy corpsman had twelve to eighteen months to train him. When doing so, the corpsman had to be aware of the concept of "face." A public comment or action to correct an error could be an unpardonable breach of respect and confidence. The corpsman had to do everything possible to draw the PF corpsman into active participation as a medic and withdraw himself from the position of an authority figure. Because of difficulty in keeping medical supplies out of the hands of the VC, the CAP corpsman was authorized to share medical supplies with the PF counterpart only for treatments that were immediately rendered in his presence.

Naval medical officers assigned to the marines also participated in medical civic action. The six doctors on the staff of "A" Medical Company, 3rd Medical Battalion, 3rd Marine Division in Da Nang, lectured on a regular basis at the Hué University Medical School, made rounds at the Provincial Hospital in Hué, and cared for orphanages and Buddhist pagodas in the region. In addition, they participated in regular medical civic action type activity in rural areas and held sick call in the base camp. In this instance, medical knowledge passed in both directions—the Dean of the Medical School, Dr. Le Khac Quyen, was a specialist in infections and tropical disease and very helpful to the American physicians.[55]

The marines attempted to establish relatively permanent

treatment facilities, rather than drop in "pill patrols." The III MAF set up programs in fixed locations and emphasized the instruction of government medical trainees. The Rural Health Workers Education Program set forth two main objectives: (1) to train a Vietnamese cadre to care for the people and (2) to produce a cadre that could train its own successors. The latter would provide for perpetuation and growth of the program.[56]

From March 1965 on, medical treatment was the most important civic action project of the Marine Corps. Only through relative permanence could training programs be established and continuity was the keynote of success.[57] The strategic position of the marines in I Corps with a geographically smaller TAOR facilitated the ability to establish relative permanency.

There were roughly ten thousand hamlets in Vietnam. If each hamlet were assigned 150 men to provide security, it would have required 1.5 million men just for that purpose. This was not feasible. If fifteen men could provide the security, when combined with indigenous local troops, it would have been feasible. The combination of U.S. forces with Vietnamese forces formed the Joint Action Company/Combined Action Company. These integrated units also provided an effective link between Free World units and the Vietnamese PF elements. To the farmers, this projected an image of equality between U.S. and Vietnamese servicemen, and this tended to counterbalance anti-U.S. sentiments.[58] This concept was the logical extension of the CAP, which functioned alone within the village or hamlet.

The need or attempt to bolster the Vietnamese health care workers while trying to teach them rather than simply rendering the aid to the people on occasion created difficulties. An outbreak of plague illustrates this conundrum well. Plague was endemic to Vietnam, occurring in twenty-seven of the forty-seven provinces in 1967.[59] There were six cases of plague in Americans who served in Vietnam, including one civilian medical technician with USAID and a case of plague meningitis in a serviceman serving with military advisors.[60] Investigation disclosed that he had not received the series of inoculations due to his movement around Vietnam.

Lt. Col. Floyd W. Baker, MC, reported on a plague outbreak in November 1967 that illustrated some of the difficulties in the MEDCAP program. A medic in an unnamed district (to avoid embarrassing the District Health Chief) learned of the possible outbreak. It would have been possible for American medical personnel to treat the patients, immunize noninfected villagers, and dust the houses with DDT to curtail the epidemic. This would not have made the Vietnamese health workers more proficient in dealing with the situation.

The involvement of the Province Health Chief's Office markedly slowed the process of controlling the epidemic. The personnel from that office were not readily available, and their investigation in the hamlet was slow. After completing their survey, they spent further time consulting with their superiors. Even more days were lost in instituting spraying and treatment. At the end of a two-week period, the Vietnamese health workers had controlled the epidemic and were in the process of teaching the village how to prevent further outbreaks.[61] It was an example of how the system was supposed to function on the one hand, but it demonstrated the difficulties in making it do so on the other.

This situation also showed the limitations of the MEDCAP program. It was designed to deliver outpatient treatments only. In reality, the coordination with the GVN was spotty at best. In some instances, there was good cooperation, and in others, the line units sent off their medical detachments with virtually no central coordination or planning. Another separate program was needed to improve the hospital care available to the Vietnamese and to upgrade the quality of hospital-based medicine. That was MILPHAP.

MILPHAP

MILPHAP, which originally stood for Military Provincial Hospital Augmentation Program, was begun in November 1965. The following year, it was redesignated as the Military Provincial Health Assistance Program (thereby retaining the same initials and creating a degree of confusion). It was under the operational control of USAID, not the military like MEDCAP. This program gained its initial impetus from President Johnson, referred to in documents as "higher authority."[62] The assistant secretary of defense instructed the three service secretaries that the teams should be "dispatched and report to Surgeon USARV soonest." (The teams actually were under the MACV Surgeon, not the USARV Surgeon.) The message authorized the secretary of the army direct liaison with the USAID to implement the program.[63] The increased participation of the military in the program occurred over the objections of USAID, which desired civilian control. This was in spite of the fact that the AID teams had been hampered by the lack of security and increasing civil strife.[64]

MILPHAP was devised to augment the civilian medical service. It was included in the 4 May 1965 message to Congress from the president, requesting additional appropriations for Vietnam.[65] MILPHAP sought to increase the service available to civilians and relieve their pain and suffering. In addition, the program hoped to portray a favorable image of the United States and its armed forces, "thereby demonstrating to the people of the Republic of Vietnam and the world that the U.S. helps people work for peace." For this reason, the uniformed MILPHAP team members stressed the fact that they were Americans or other FWMAF personnel.[66] It was also to show the civilian populace that the GVN and ARVN were deeply interested in their welfare,[67] though exactly how emphasizing that the care being rendered by foreigners in their military uniforms accomplished this remains unclear.

Initially, MILPHAP placed a sixteen-man U.S. or other

FWMAF team in each of the forty-three civilian province hospitals. These teams sought to upgrade the quality and quantity of medical inpatient support available to Vietnamese civilians. As hospital-based teams dealing with inpatients, MILPHAP teams were prohibited from MEDCAP missions by regulation.[68] They worked under the direction of the province medical chief, who was recognized as an "individual of stature, medically as well as politically."[69]

The developing MEDCAP II program, related to the U.S. troop buildup, could accomplish the tasks desired of the mobile medical teams.[70] Its expansion with the utilization of the additional personnel in country and medical sections organic to line units would not have truly improved the health care of the rural Vietnamese, though it would make limited outpatient care more widely available. It was decided that supporting and augmenting the USOM/USAID Provincial Health Assistance Program by providing surgical teams would attain the best results. This was the beginning of the MILPHAP concept.[71]

The MILPHAP mission was to provide medical care and health services to Vietnamese civilians, train hospital staff workers, and develop the surgical skills of the Vietnamese physicians.  Due to a shortage of trained surgeons available to the program, volunteer U.S. civilian surgeons augmented the program through Project Vietnam.[72] Financed by USAID and sponsored by the American Medical Association, it supplied physicians who served sixty-day tours in a Vietnamese provincial hospital. The volunteers worked with Vietnamese medical and health personnel to augment, develop, and expand Vietnamese capabilities in clinical health care and public health programs at the district and village/hamlet level. By September 1971, efforts and staffing were directed primarily toward training the local personnel in preventive medicine and public health.[73]

MILPHAP team commanders did not assume responsibility for the operation of a provincial hospital or health service but were expected to assist and support the province medical chief in carrying out his responsibilities for the health measures within the province. The civilian province medical chief remained in charge and had veto power over U.S. team proposals. MILPHAP team members used persuasion and demonstrations to obtain the reforms necessary to establish an efficient medical service. This process was hampered by a lack of understanding of the cultural differences between American and Vietnamese in regard to criticism and public correction.[74] As Henry Kissinger noted, it would be difficult to imagine two societies less meant to understand each other than the Vietnamese and American.[75]

In late 1967 there were twenty-two MILPHAP teams in country: eight army, seven air force, and seven navy.[76] Each team consisted of three medical officers, a medical administrative officer, eleven enlisted medical technicians, and an enlisted administrative specialist. The teams brought equipment into Vietnam supplied through U.S. military channels. According to a joint MACV/USOM directive, the COMUSMACV was responsible for logistical and administrative support. USAID funded all expendable medical supplies. The USOM director was responsible for supplying drivers and interpreters. As is readily apparent, this organizational structure meant that the team had to supply its needs from multiple sources and therefore was forced to deal with multiple logistical and administrative structures.[77]

MILPHAP teams made a substantial direct contribution to the improvement of hospitalization capability in Vietnam. The teams also provided an organized infrastructure that could be used by individual volunteer physicians, nurses, technicians, and other health workers from the United States and other assistance programs. The success of the MILPHAP concept was attested to by the fact that other free world nations deployed similar teams to Vietnam, both military and civilian.[78]

Despite MILPHAP's accomplishments, its institutional structure was an organizational nightmare. According to the military, the "command and administrative arrangements for MILPHAP teams were poorly defined. The Commander USMACV, USAID, and the USOM all shared control of MILPHAP."[79] Personnel, supplies, and logistical support came from various entities.

There was an ongoing problem with such basic considerations as vehicle maintenance since there were no mechanics attached to the units. In a cumbersome arrangement, motor vehicle maintenance was provided by ARVN units arranged by MACV and drivers were Vietnamese provided by the embassy.[80] The vehicles themselves came from USARV (the logistical side of the command). As late as 1970, one MILPHAP team reported being without a radio for a year and without telephone service on multiple occasions for up to ten weeks.[81] USARV provided supply support for the teams in II, III, and IV Corps, while Naval Support Activity (NSA) Da Nang supported the I Corps teams. Command and control were under MACV through the MACV surgeon.

The time-limited tour in Vietnam also presented a problem for MILPHAP. Initially, the original groups or teams were trained and formed as a unit in the United States and then deployed in Vietnam. It was planned to replace the team *in toto* with a new team, but it readily became apparent that this would not work well. Difficulties in the timing of arrival of replacements resulted in either overlap between the teams or a hiatus in operations, undermining the goal of continuity. Further, replacing an entire team caused a loss of institutional memory, meaning that the entire learning process had to begin anew. MACV soon deemed it necessary to switch to an individual member replacement policy to avoid replacing an entire team at one time. (The navy did continue to utilize the concept of team replacement.)[82]

MILPHAP had the best chance of all the medical programs to make a long-term difference and improvement in the Vietnamese health care system. To a great extent, the program was oriented toward teaching, with the potential for the development of permanent benefits. As with many aspects of the war, there was often a conflict between the U.S. personnel wanting to get the task done quickly and properly as opposed to having their Vietnamese counterparts do it. Teaching under these circumstances was difficult, as SSG Terry Hammes of the 447th Medical Detachment in Pleiku commented, "We frequently push the Vietnamese into the background because we do not feel that they are doing as good a job as they should be doing."[83] MILPHAP never received the publicity that MEDCAP did and was far less likely to be the focus of stories in the domestic U.S. press.

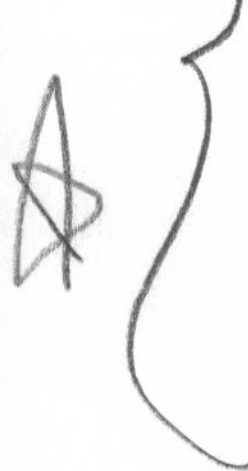

MEDCAP, MILPHAP, the PHAP, and AGHD organizations were all intended to deliver medical care to civilians, without consideration of the types of medical need or their causes. MEDCAP I and II were rudimentary outpatient primary care programs; MILPHAP upgraded hospital care, including surgical specialties and increased the availability of these treatments to the population. None of these programs specifically addressed the needs of civilians injured in the war. The Civilian War Casualty Program (CWCP) did so.

CWCP

Significant disagreements regarding the number of South Vietnamese civilian casualties during the war remain to this day. Some patients were erroneously categorized as war casualties and others were reported twice when they were transferred from a GVN to a U.S. military hospital or vice versa.[84] In some instances, the type of injury led to erroneous classification as a war-related injury. Flight surgeon Capt. Gerald McGowan reported seeing eight to ten burn patients a day. Many of these cases resulted from using purloined jet fuel as household fuel. A report by the Children's Medical Relief International, Inc., found that 85 percent of the burn cases in the hospitals were from civilian (not war-related) causes.[85] If the interpreters were not adequate to determine an accurate history, many of these cases could have appeared to be due to napalm burns, which was simply inaccurate. Hospital admissions for civilian napalm burns were actually a rarity,[86] in part because the patients did not live to get to the hospital.

Some organizations sought to use the civilian casualties to embarrass the United States. The Swiss-based *Terre Des Hommes* claimed there were "numerous seriously or fatally burned or wounded children" that could be saved by being evacuated from Vietnam to hospitals in Europe and that they were "dying like flies in Kontum Hospital because of lack of medicines." The U.S. position (and that of the GVN) was that they should be treated in Vietnam. Their allegations of inadequate treatment and a refusal by the United States to allow them to help were repeated by the British Vietnam Committee. A subsequent visit by a *Terre Des Hommes* supervisory nurse, Miss E. Darbre, refuted these allegations, noting that the high mortality rates were due to climatic conditions, unhygienic conditions, and only incidentally to lack of a few recently developed medicines.[87] As is often the case, the "correction" received far less media attention than the original accusations.

Arguments persist about whether these casualties were due to U.S. and FWMAF actions or to those of the VC and NVA. Many military leaders criticized the media for emphasizing casualties caused by U.S. bombing and artillery, but ignoring those caused by the VC and NVA, especially after Tet in 1968 and the accompanying massacres of civilians, as in Hué. Senator Edward Kennedy (D-MA) arbitrarily chose to double the military figures for casualties and hospital admissions. He did not believe the United States was assuming sufficient responsibility for the civilian casualty and refugee problem in Vietnam.[88]

The Kennedy team was upset to see patients lying on the floor in some instances, and multiple patients in a bed in others. Lying on sweaty linens in bed is more uncomfortable than upon a dry mat on the floor, especially if one is used to sleeping on a mat over a hard surface. Further, in the absence of air conditioning, the floor was cooler. As discussed previously, it was normal and most comfortable for most Vietnamese to sleep with others in a bed, and they were often uncomfortable if made to stay in a bed alone. Parents may have demanded to stay in the same bed with a sick child so that he or she would not be afraid.[89]

The same data could lead to very different conclusions about the meaning of civilian casualties. Senator Kennedy stated that security in Vietnam had not improved because civilian war casualties in 1970 ran at about the same rate as in 1967. On the other hand, the Saigon Embassy and the State Department interpreted this data to mean that security had improved to the point where a higher percentage of casualties could reach the hospital. Therefore, the same number of patients reaching the hospital implied a lower casualty rate.[90] For perspective, through March 1968, it was estimated that approximately 150,000 South Vietnamese civilians had been injured as a result of hostilities. A total of 4,799 civilian war casualties were treated in U.S. military hospitals during the period 1 January 1967 to 20 May 1968.[91] Secretary of State Dean Rusk acknowledged the impossibility to accurately know the number of war-related injuries not receiving treatment, especially in remote areas, or those caused by the enemy.[92]

The important question of which side caused the casualties was difficult to answer. Injuries from mines, booby traps, punji stakes, etc., were considered enemy-inflicted because friendly forces did not use those weapons. Injuries from small arms fire were listed as questionable, as both sides used these weapons. Injuries resulting from artillery or air strikes were listed as due to friendly fire.[93] Medical personnel in the theater attributed about 40 percent of civilian casualties to enemy acts, 30 percent to small arms or mortar fire that could have come from either side, and 30 percent to friendly artillery or aerial bombardment based on the type of injuries that they saw. Applying this estimate to the 4,000 civilian casualties per month, about 1,600 can be attributed to the enemy. If the GVN/FWMAF accepted blame for the remaining casualties, they would be responsible for 2,400 per month. This analysis, however, underestimates the casualties caused by enemy action. They deliberately used terror as a tactic, employing grenades, land mines, and booby traps. For example, the VC shelled populated areas indiscriminately and deliberately drew air strikes upon a village by firing on aircraft, then fleeing when the hamlet or village came under attack. If half of the nonattributed 30 percent of casualties were due to enemy actions, then the NVA/VC was responsible for some 2,200 per month and the FWMAF was responsible for 1,800.[94] Obviously, these estimates are somewhat arbitrary.

A 1971 USAID letter to Senator Kennedy reported statistics obtained from the Vietnamese MOH. They reported 184,515 civilian war casualties admitted to GVN hospitals from 1967 to 1969, of which 79,653 (about 42 percent) were caused by mines and mortar fire and thus attributed to the enemy, 64,334 (about 35 percent) by shelling and bombing and attributed to the allies, and 40,528 (22 percent) by guns and grenades, which might have been caused by either side. They also noted trends in that the proportion of casualties caused by mines and mortars was on the rise, those from guns and grenades remained fairly steady, and those from bombing and shelling were decreasing.[95]

General Westmoreland recognized the implication of massive civilian war casualties to the war effort. In a 1965 MACV directive, he noted that "the use of unnecessary force leading to noncombatant battle casualties in areas temporarily controlled by the VC will embitter the population, drive them into the arms of the VC, and make the long-range goal of pacification more difficult and more costly."[96] These circumstances required restraint not normally demanded of soldiers on the battlefield. Elimination of harassment and interdiction (H&I) fire-support missions was intended to decrease the number of civilian casualties.[97] The directive further noted that the VC exploited incidents of noncombatant casualties with the objective of fostering resentment against the GVN and the United States.

At a time when there was growing public debate over U.S. foreign policy in Vietnam, it was politically expedient to emphasize the humanitarian aspects of U.S. involvement.[98] MACV had a policy to actively assist in treating civilian war casualties from the beginning of the 1965 buildup of U.S. troops.[99] Care of civilians in U.S. military hospitals on an emergency basis had been authorized from the beginning of the American troop buildup.[100]

In an effort to quell the furor over civilian casualties, on 16 August 1967, Secretary of Defense Robert McNamara announced the construction of three hospitals with 1,100 beds for Vietnamese civilians who had suffered war-related injuries.[101] Congressman Porter Hardy accused the administration of "knuckling under" to Senator Kennedy and constructing hospitals that were not needed,[102] as there had never been a shortage of beds for civilians. The hospitals were to be built at Da Nang and Chu Lai, as well as in the Mekong Delta, most likely at Can Tho. They were to be for civilian use only.

While these hospitals would have created a highly visible program with maximum publicity, they would not have provided the greatest amount of hospital support to the greatest number of people, the ostensible objective of the program. Since casualties were occurring throughout the country, transportation problems would have been significant with that construction program. Furthermore, many South Vietnamese were reluctant to leave their own provinces due to the religious belief that if one dies outside his or her own province, the soul wanders forever in a lost state.[103] The absence of adequate nurses compelled many Vietnamese families to accompany the sick or injured to the hospital to provide care, creating even more transportation difficulties. Instead of building more hospitals, the United States concluded that a more reasonable approach was to share occupancy in the already existing U.S. forces hospital system in Vietnam. For these reasons, the visibility that the program would have achieved with specially designated hospitals was sacrificed to provide better care.[104] It was recognized within the White House that the change to augmenting existing hospitals rather than building new, specially dedicated hospitals would cause displeasure.[105]

By May 1968, the DOD had approved the policy of joint utilization with the anticipation that treating patients closer to their homes would reduce transportation requirements and the number of family members arriving at the hospital with each patient. At no time following the 1968 Tet offensive was bed space in MACV hospitals a significant factor limiting care of civilians.[106] From July 1969 onward, admissions of civilians to MACV hospitals decreased as the joint utilization program of the Vietnamese Ministry of Health and the ARVN became increasingly capable of caring for injured civilians.[107] This enabled MACV to steadily decrease the number of beds allotted to the CWCP from 1,100 in 1968 to 200 by 1971.[108]

Most of the Vietnamese people, especially in rural areas, attached great importance to dying at home and being buried near the village. Many villages prohibited the transportation of corpses. Therefore, when a patient was critically ill or worsened in the hospital, the family often took him home to be near the home burial ground.[109]

Emergency medical care to Vietnamese nationals in U.S. military hospitals was authorized to prevent undue suffering or loss of life when Vietnamese medical care was not readily available. Such cases were to be transferred to the nearest GVN treatment facility as soon as medically feasible. Dr. Howard Rusk, president of the World Rehabilitation Fund, considered the establishment of hospitals to treat civilian war casualties a historic milestone: "Never before in history has any nation in the world established a military operated hospital program in wartime to care for injured civilians."[110] Statistical data showed the success of the program. From June 1964 through December 1968, 69,590 civilians were admitted as inpatients to U.S. Army hospitals for total bed occupancy of 246,010 days. An additional 788,472 civilians were seen as outpatients at the hospitals.[111]

MACV Directive 40-14 (10 January 1968) authorized medical treatment for Vietnamese nationals in U.S. medical facilities only on a space available basis, and such treatment "was not to detract from the primary mission of the medical facility." Further, specialized medical or surgical treatment would be given only when this type of treatment was unavailable through normal Vietnamese medical channels. The furnishing of such care "must enhance the mission of U.S. Army, Vietnam" and was contingent on approval by the commanding general, USARV, for each individual case. Change 1 to this directive the following year authorized treatment of personnel employed by the US/FWMAF as Kit Carson or Tiger Scouts (Vietnamese soldiers and former VC cadre members working for the U.S. military) for complete medical services for "occupational injuries." Again, once the scout's medical condition was stabilized, he or she was to be transferred to the nearest GVN civilian treatment facility. RVN civilians were not to be admitted for care of chronic diseases, psychiatric conditions, or conditions with a known poor prognosis (unless the condition was war related).[112]

By 1972, the GVN medical system was capable of handling the civilian war casualty patient load, in spite of the Easter Offensive by the North.[113] It was no longer necessary to maintain 200-bed availability within the U.S. system to support the CWCP, but it was changed to a policy of providing support on a case by case basis within existing capabilities. This change enabled the U.S. hospitals to provide the needed services in the face of the continued draw down of U.S. forces.

The various programs provided varying types of health care in different settings to the people of Vietnam. There was a primary care traveling program (MEDCAP), a hospital-based program to train and deliver more complex and sophisticated care (MIL-

PHAP), and a program to care for the war-related injuries to the people (CWCP). It would be gratifying to believe they were interrelated and provided a comprehensive system of health care to the Vietnamese, served to gain the friendship and support of the people, and weaned the rural population away from the enemy and into the arms of the government of South Vietnam. The next two chapters will assess the programs' success in delivering satisfactory medical care and fulfilling U.S. policy aims.

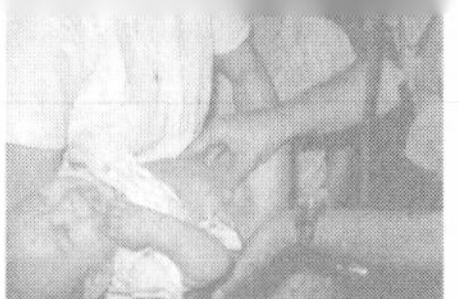

Five
Medical Evaluation of the Programs

There are at least two major aspects of these programs to evaluate: the medical care provided and the use of the various programs to implement policy. The first of these will be discussed in this chapter and the second in the next. While the two areas are not mutually exclusive, they do not necessarily coincide or overlap and the assessment of the programs may well differ when the two aspects are examined. One must also bear in mind that the medical assessments were made by those "in the field," whereas the policy evaluations emanated from the command level.

Before evaluating MEDCAP, it is useful to look at the manner in which the program was actually conducted. Often the reality "on the ground" differed significantly from the planning on paper. How the plans and programs were carried out in reality bears significantly upon any evaluation.

If the end of the war raised doubts about the usefulness of the civilian care to the war effort, there had been much support generated for the program's value just a few months earlier. The focus was on acquiring support for the effort on the home front. During the peak American military involvement in Vietnam, 1966 to 1970, the army, navy, and marines disseminated a plethora of anecdotal MEDCAP reports intended to generate favorable publicity for the program and cast the U.S. military in a favorable light. These stories appeared in many hometown newspapers,[1] as well as military publications as *Army,*[2] *Army Reporter,*[3] *Army Digest,*[4] *U.S. Navy Medicine,*[5] *Marine Corps Gazette,*[6] *Airman,*[7] and unit newspapers.[8] While they provided good human interest stories and favorable press for the military, they were of little value in evaluating the quality of medical care or the significance of the programs to the war effort.

Statements found in *The Screaming Eagle,* the paper of the 101st Airborne Division, were typical of such accounts: "A MEDCAP team of the 101st Airborne entered a small fishing village southwest of here recently, accepting the initial cool reception and leaving six hours later with the gratitude and friendship of the villagers."[9] This report, pertaining to a single MEDCAP mission by recounting the one-day team experience of the paratroopers of the 2nd Battalion, 327th Infantry and giving the names and hometowns of the corpsmen and the battalion surgeon, would be easily reprinted in a hometown newspaper. Generous conclusions regarding the feelings of the villagers after one short visit were drawn in the short piece from little information and no data.

The unit reports of MEDCAP activities were similarly flawed. They only provided generalizations about the care rendered or the numbers of patients treated. For example, Advisory Team 100 simply stated that "the medical civic action program continues to be highly effective with large numbers of civilians treated throughout the Hop Tac area."[10] As Lt. Col. Peter B. Cramblet, MSC, cautioned in his War College paper on medicine in low intensity conflicts, "Exercises that accumulate impressive statistics for patients treated are a meaningless method of management by body count."[11] The reporting in the news media and military publications was highly anecdotal and intended to be laudatory rather than unbiased reporting. Therefore, it is apparent that determining the true record of the programs as well as evaluating their impact is difficult. It is only by amassing many unit reports and yearly summaries over time and throughout the country that a full picture can be obtained.

Tracing the experience of the 11th Armored Cavalry (AC) Regiment, which arrived in Vietnam in the fall of 1966, provides a sample of the reports over an extended time. By following the trail of civic action activities in the Operational Reports from the fall of 1966 to the winter of 1970, a picture develops of their activities.[12] On 31 October 1966, the short paragraph dealing with civil affairs states, "One MEDCAP mission was accomplished in the Phu Hoi village, which treated 70 civilians. It is noteworthy that Phu Hoi has been a VC dominated village for several years." The next report (5 December 1966) notes that only twenty people "permitted the MEDCAP team to administer any medical aid." It appeared that the people had been indoctrinated by the VC to the "dire consequences" of accepting help from the U.S. troops.

By the end of January 1967, more than a thousand Vietnamese were receiving medical aid from the regiment, primarily for respiratory disorders and dietary deficiencies. A total of 1,565 patients were examined and treated in April 1967, most frequently for anemia and URI-otic (ear) disease in children. Intelligence was gleaned from ralliers and individuals treated during MEDCAPs.

A July 1967 report comments that "the regiment's emphasis on MEDCAP showed positive results as the number of patients treated increased fourfold. A total of 299,971 patients were treated. In addition, thirty-five patients were treated during DENTCAPS." The only other evaluation equates an increase in number of people treated with progress, analogous to citing increased body counts with progress toward winning the war.

Some programs clashed with the cultural or religious mores of the country. While rabies was a significant problem with more than seven hundred cases reported in 1968, according to Wallis Craddock (Col., MC), there was no rabies control program in the country as the Buddhist religion "posed a barrier" due to the prohibition on the destruction of dogs and other animals.[13] The U.S. Veterinary Corps worked vigorously to institute a rabies control program, both as part of the civic action programs and to immunize and protect the animals many servicemen adopted as pets. This benefited both the Vietnamese and the U.S. forces.

Visits by medical brigade personnel to combat units illustrated the differences in viewpoints about the MEDCAP programs. The 11th AC regimental surgeon and the doctors in the medical company who felt pressured into uncoordinated activities to "look good" on the charts and graphs were disenchanted with MEDCAP. On the other hand, the unit executive officer spoke enthusiastically about the program and emphasized its importance. He was unaware of the comments made by his own doctors.[14]

Certain trends and tendencies occur throughout these reports filed over almost five years. Numbers were used to show the state of the program, with absolutely no commentary regarding the quality of medicine delivered to the people. There was a recurring theme pertaining to the usefulness of the program in obtaining intelligence. This intelligence dealt primarily with locations and movements of local small enemy units, ambushes, and booby traps. The tactical situation was reflected with decreasing activity in the program during periods of heightened military activity as in Tet 1968 and the increased needs of the population after the battles were over. Some units reported no assistance to civilians whatsoever in the period of the Tet offensives.[15]

Other units filed similar reports. In the 1st Infantry Division Operational Report for the period 1 May to 31 July 1966, under the MEDCAP heading was the following paragraph: "The Division MEDCAP Program has expanded to support the dependents of the ARVN 5th Division. The MEDCAP activities conducted in conjunction with the LAM SON Operation can account for the treatment of over 27,000 patients of the 59,000 total for the division. The large increase over the previous report is primarily due to the introduction of LAM SON II. MEDCAP continues to be conducted in conjunction with all division operations plus the normal treatment around base camp areas."[16]

The obviously rounded-off numbers make their inclusion in a statistical evaluation dubious at best. These large numbers were generated by counting the extensive vaccination programs as well as more routine medical visits. There was no other evaluation of the program.

The 1st Air Cavalry Division listed their MEDCAP objectives as follows: (1) to develop and maintain a friendly relationship between the members of the division and the population within the TAOR, (2) to improve the general level of health within the Division area, (3) to train health workers where needed, and (4) to develop dispensaries that become an asset and responsibility of the Vietnamese. The division began a nurse training program in Son Tan village with twelve Vietnamese women and began a similar program in An Son. In an interesting note, the MEDCAPs in Cun An [*sic*] and San An were carried out in conjunction with the Korean MEDCAP program.[17]

In the 11th Combat Aviation Battalion report for 1 May to 31 July 1966, is the statement that MEDCAP had been carried out by all medical units within the battalion. All of the medical units held sick call for Vietnamese nationals using medical supplies obtained through MEDCAP. Most of the patients seen were young children or elderly people. "The average number of patients seen is about 95 per visit. Approximately 8 visits are conducted per month by this battalion's medical personnel."[18] Some reports were even less quantified, as that of the 3rd Field Hospital, which states, "The MEDCAP effort at the 3rd Field Hospital has been directed at establishing sound medical out-patient care for Vietnamese civilians and at improving medical care at existing Vietnamese medical facilities. In general the program has been successful and well received by the Vietnamese."[19] Generalizations and approximations abound in the reports. No attempt was made to evaluate the program in any meaningful manner, and there is no substantiation for the conclusions reached.

The 58th Medical Battalion Army Medical Service Activities Report for the year of 1968 noted the fluctuation of MEDCAP activity with the tactical situation. Further, included within the number of patients treated were "Local Nationals" who worked on the post. While their medical care was beneficial to them, it did not advance the effort to gain support of the population. Total patient numbers ranged from a low of 2,200 in March to 6,900 in April. The yearly total was "approximately" 40,000.[20]

The 9th Infantry reported a total of 160 MEDCAPs held during 1968. A total of 15,510 patients were seen and treated in the "formal Medcap plan of the battalion." There was also the comment that "in addition to the formal (Medcap) programs the company aidmen held informal medcaps in the various company areas of operation." No numbers were given for those activities. No discussion of the difference between the formal and casual programs is contained in the report. The report concluded, "These programs have been contributing significantly to area pacification,"[21] without citing any basis for this conclusion.

The 1st Battalion, 5th Infantry averaged anywhere from zero to eight MEDCAPs per week, treating from fifteen to 3,600 on each MEDCAP. That unusually large last figure was due to a plague epidemic in the village of Trung Lap. The battalion medics immunized approximately 3,600 people in one day. The battalion surgeon treated twenty plague victims per day.[22]

Other reports are totally devoid of any quantification. For instance, the 4th Battalion, 23rd Infantry (MECH), 25th Division report stated that MEDCAPs were conducted daily. "An attempt is made to inculcate into the local areas a sense of personal hygiene and public health. Villages are visited on a weekly basis whenever possible." Vietnamese nurses and civilians were encouraged to participate in the treatment of patients. This was done by "turning over the cleaning and bandaging of 'cuts' and 'bruises' to one who shows interest" and then teaching them how to care for the patients. The last notation was that "all patients who seem to be sick are seen by the Battalion Surgeon who is present at all MEDCAPs."[23]

The 2nd Battalion, 34th Armor of the 25th Division provided

screening of indigenous personnel working in the mess halls at base camp, an activity more to the benefit of the U.S. troops than to the aid of the indigenous population. MEDCAPs were held "about once a week" with "approximately 2,000 Vietnamese treated in July, August, and the first few days of September." Problems with the MEDCAP program were noted with the supply system: "Due to the fact we have not received an account number to entitle us to requisition MEDCAP supplies, our supplies are obtained from the 173rd Airborne Brigade in Bien Hoa."[24]

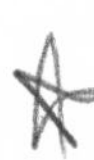

The 2/34 Armor and 5/2 Artillery, 25th Division units saw the patients in their aid stations, rather than going into the villages. Lack of adequate security hampered the program, and ARVN, RF, and PF support was haphazard. At times, they would not appear, and at other times, they would "wander off" when they were supposed to be providing ongoing protection in the field.[25] More complete treatment was available in the aid station than on visits to the hamlets, and the U.S. personnel wasted less time. They had people come into the base camp aid station because, (1) inadequate treatment was sometimes worse than no treatment and (2) people motivated enough to seek care for themselves or others too ill to come into the aid station are better and more grateful patients.

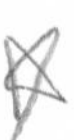

Reporting of MEDCAP activity ranged from the nonspecific "a great number of patients have been treated"[26] to a table provided in the 2nd Battalion, 22nd Infantry report giving a monthly detail of the number of MEDCAPs and patients seen for the year.[27] This last report included the statement that "generally all MEDCAP projects were quite successful in that a great deal of medical aid and medical supplies were dispensed to the local populous [*sic*] who are always enthusiastic in their gratitude." The number of people seen and the amount of medicines dispensed served as the measure of the program, with no attempt to measure medical efficacy. In another report, after stating that sick calls were made twice weekly with sanitary measures stressed at each visit, there was the more cautious statement that "some improvement in the health and hygiene of the individuals in the village was noted."[28]

With virtually every combat unit in country carrying out MEDCAP activities, many more such reports could be cited with no particular increase in knowledge about the programs. While they tend to be highly anecdotal, a pattern does emerge as multiple such reports are reviewed.

Many, if not most, of the conclusions within the reports are totally without supporting documentation. They are replete with generalizations, unsubstantiated impressions, and baseless conclusions regarding the effect they have had on the indigenous population and its relationship or regard for the American troops. It is not possible to either give full credence to these conclusions or have a basis for discrediting them.

The reality of the hamlet MEDCAP carried out on the battalion or small unit level is not completely reflected in these reports. Frequently, there was little or no coordination with the district health officials, beyond receiving permission to go into a specific hamlet. In many instances, the visits were unannounced to avoid ambushes. In my personal experience, there was no contact between the GVN and the medical unit. Permission was given to the unit commander to go into a village without coordination with the local dispensary or hospital facility, or other units operating in the same area. The MEDCAP team, with its security detail, would enter the hamlet and set up shop in a school or dispensary. In our case, security was provided by our own battalion. There were no Vietnamese medical workers involved in the MEDCAPs. The people would learn by word of mouth that the doctor, or *bac si,* was visiting. It could take weeks of effort to surmount the initial distrust of Westerners. Mainly children and the elderly were seen, as the young adults were either in the army or working in the fields. Over one eight-month period, the Medical Civic Action Team 20 operating near Da-nang reported 45 percent of the patients seen were children, and 39 percent were women.[29]

Lt. Col. Joseph R. Territo, the programs officer in the USARV Surgeon's Office, warned against becoming involved in "traveling circuses." While tactical MEDCAPs were necessary, a one-time visit accomplished nothing and was viewed as a "shot-gun approach" and not good medicine. A good MEDCAP was a recurring activity on a scheduled basis and provided for patient follow-up. It is obvious that this was difficult if security concerns limited or prevented scheduled return visits. It was also important to involve the local health care workers.[30]

Capt. John Irving (Armor) described a MEDCAP mission as a military maneuver. "The small column moved out of the main gate, down the dirt road through the deserted rubber plantation, in a swirl of dust. Abruptly, the four *M113* armed personnel carriers (APCs) swung off the road and entered a small hamlet of twenty to thirty mud huts. The APCs moved rapidly to the left and right edges of the village, while the remainder of the column, two-ton trucks and an *M577* medical vehicle, huddled near the center."[31] Whether this "invasion" aided in winning the hearts and minds of the villagers is an open question.

The language barrier persisted as a significant problem. In most U.S. military units there were no Vietnamese speaking personnel. The ability of the team to treat was limited by the quality of the available interpreters. Both civilian and ARVN military interpreters were utilized. Their effectiveness varied greatly and markedly improved as they assisted on more MEDCAPs. This was especially true if one interpreter could work with one medical unit for a significant length of time. A change in the TAOR of the unit frequently resulted in new interpreters being assigned to work with the team, thus restarting the learning process. It was extremely difficult to obtain medical histories through an interpreter, especially if he or she were untrained in the field of medicine. This difficulty was compounded when working through a chain of interpreters, as a Vietnamese interpreter going through a Montagnard or Hmong tribesman. The result of this deficiency was extremely sketchy medical histories, and consequently, basically symptomatic treatments being given to the patients.[32]

Most line units participating in the MEDCAP program did not keep any medical records of the Vietnamese patients treated. In view of the absence of laboratory or radiological capability, treatment was based solely on the medical history given and physical diagnosis. Treatments for illnesses were oriented toward short-term cure, rather than long-term programs for the treatments of diseases such as tuberculosis or malaria. The experience of most MEDCAP doctors convinced them that the majority of patient complaints were due to chronic problems that could neither be diagnosed nor treated in a single visit. There was a tendency to fall back to symptomatic treatment of immediate complaints.[33]

It was important that every patient be given something, be it medicine or soap. One report commented that while the program is "of limited value medically, it is an outstanding tool for propaganda."[34] Another battalion surgeon complained about "the inability to have long term follow-up, and a lack of laboratory facilities for definitive diagnosis and treatment."[35]

Line units "MEDCAPed" on a regular basis, at least weekly. This did not mean the return to the same hamlet on a regular basis. Due to security considerations, in many instances, return visits could not be announced or scheduled in advance for fear of ambush (though in view of the very few attacks on MEDCAP teams, this fear was most likely exaggerated). Since follow-up medical care was sporadic and unpredictable, it was difficult, if not impossible, to sustain long-term treatment of chronic diseases. Even during the conflict, MEDCAP teams realized that inadequate treatment resulted from one-time visits, no follow-up treatment, and crowded and nonfunctional MEDCAP areas.[36]

Naval units participated in tactical MEDCAP activities as well. The navy also provided the physicians and corpsmen assigned to marine units. Civic action materials were obtained in part from CARE, USAID, and the Catholic Relief Organization for distribution.[37] Landing Ship Medical (LSM) 400 hospital ships (medium landing craft fitted for medical care) treated villagers and those living on small islands while making their rounds. In May 1966, one ship treated 4,400 people, including four hundred dental patients and twenty minor surgery cases, during an eleven-day period. Children with cleft lip deformity were operated on, and one blind child had her eyes replaced with artificial eyes "to cosmetically improve her appearance." First aid was administered to Vietnamese civilians aboard junks encountered during board and search operations.[38]

More seriously ill patients or patients with tumors beyond the capability of the team to manage in the field were referred to the nearest Vietnamese treatment facility, generally the provincial hospital. There was no system to ensure that the patients actually went to the hospital and received treatment. Again, this was a function of the absence of a medical record or a routine system of follow-up. Unfortunately, many rural peasants feared the world outside their village, and patients who were told they would require hospitalization might disappear.[39] Ideally, a local village health provider would have been present at all MEDCAPs to administrate and follow-up on these situations, but that was not always the case and, in fact, was actually quite unusual. Without medical records or an ability to recall patients, feedback to the MEDCAP team was nonexistent.

As the 1st Battalion, 12th Cavalry put it, "The nature of operation in Vietnam results in frequent contact with indigenous personnel." This provided the medical platoon with "abundant opportunities" to treat civilians, often done on an informal basis and without the battalion surgeon. These informal sick calls not only provided medical care to many areas for the first time, but also eased the fears of civilians in the combat area. Combat operations ended with a civic action team entering the village to hold sick call and gain information. The minor ailments were treated in place and attempts were made to evacuate seriously ill civilians to provincial hospitals.[40] Generally, the number of individuals treated medically during maneuvers was unreported.

In addition to providing medical care, the program also supplied important medical intelligence. It provided a picture of the general health of the indigenous population. Common problems encountered included vitamin deficiencies, respiratory diseases, intestinal disorders, and dermatological problems associated with inadequate personal hygiene. "Unfortunately the vast majority of disorders could only be remedied but not cured." Follow-up treatment was possible in only a few villages.[41] Frequently injectable antibiotics were used to prevent pills and liquid medicines falling into enemy hands.[42]

The advantages of the same unit remaining in one location for a prolonged period of time are obvious. Perversely, the best results were therefore achieved in a locale where the program was least needed, one of relative stability and allegiance to the GVN. If one aim of the various programs was to build support for the GVN, effectiveness in areas already supporting it made little difference. The experience of the 1st Howitzer Battery, 40th Artillery was exemplary. U.S. military and Vietnamese civilians constructed a village aid station with a concrete floor and tin covered wooden frame. Weekly patient visits were made with "rewarding and encouraging" follow-up care. A general improvement in the health of villagers occurred, according to those participating in the program and submitting the report. There is no data available for any evaluation of these statements regarding significant alterations or improvements in the health of the village, and they must simply be taken as the impressions of those who were there. A partially trained Vietnamese aidman participated in the conduct of the MEDCAP, and efforts were made to further educate him.[43] The abandoned French hospital in Dong Ha was reconstructed the following year with supplies obtained in part from private U.S. donations, with the expectation that routine MEDCAP supply channels would maintain the facility.

Other units in the locale also participated in the hospital reconstruction project.[44] One year later, the unit was still supporting the hospital with medical support for both inpatient and outpatient services.

It is impossible to evaluate a program without recognizing its goals. Unfortunately, even the military was unclear in this regard. The MAAG report on the programs noted that "confusion continued on the U.S. side concerning the ultimate objective of the program: the medical relief of suffering or the political winning of the civilian population. The two poles of thought supported different operational methods."[45] Comparison studies of different MEDCAP visit methods were not done "since it would require after-action studies of the attitudes of the various village populations."[46] Col. Raymond Bishop Jr., MC, in his War College study of the programs in Vietnam, maintains that the military remained confused in this regard.[47]

While the two possible objectives are similar and overlap, the implementation and emphasis would vary depending on which choice was considered primary. If the primary objective was to improve the health of the people and relieve their suffering, then a "bonus effect" is that the people will become grateful to the Republic of Vietnam for providing this care and might support the government. If the primary objective is to win the confidence and loyalty of the people, a "bonus effect" from this is that it might improve their health and relative suffering.[48]

When the medical effort is admittedly a vehicle to achieve part of a military goal, civic action or psychological warfare officers have operational control rather than U.S. medical advisors. In such an arrangement, it is not surprising that MEDCAP doctors felt insufficient attention was paid to the actual treatment needs and that their contribution was merely a "medicine show" designed to attract a crowd. Overall, as shown in the medical activities reports, doctors felt that the medical discipline was being prostituted for a less worthy purpose. On the other hand, if the primary objective was to relieve suffering and improve the health of the people, emphasis would be on preventive medicine and education in hygiene and sanitation, as well as training of local health workers. Doctors would have a major and significant role. If the primary objective was to impress the rural population and win them over to support the government, there was no need for a doctor to go on every village visit.

There was virtually uniform agreement among physicians that single-visit, drop-in, unplanned, and uncoordinated MEDCAP visits were of negligible medical value, at best. Many reports contain phrases as, "I am convinced that fly-by-night Med CAPS, without the approval and support of the local Vietnamese health officials, do more harm than good to the U.S. Army and the Republic of Vietnam."[49] Another said, "I think that most of us who were doing the MEDCAPing realized after 10 or 15 of these MEDCAPs, or probably realized after one of them, that this was not a very productive long range program."[50] Lowell Rubin, medical corps officer with the 4th Infantry Division, found that MEDCAP visits were based on very limited contact. Long-term objectives were overlooked, and in large part, the good accomplished ceased when the visits ceased.[51] An end-of-tour report noted that "MEDCAP is one of the outstanding goodwill pacification programs available. It is a poor medical program."[52] One battalion surgeon described the therapeutic value of the program as negligible, "with the single exception being the case of infectious diseases especially as seen in the pediatric age group."[53] Another Medical Services Activities Report described the program as "of limited value medically, but an outstanding tool for propaganda."[54] A 23rd Division (Americal) Medical Service Activities Report contained the following sentence: "The main complaint of this facility concerning MEDCAPs is that they cannot be done on a regular basis thus allowing a follow-up to be made on patients treated."[55]

Medical Corps Lt. Col. Chas. Webb described the "sick-call patrol" as a high impact short-range program.[56] In many cases, less medicine is practiced than "medical show business." The medic or doctor who sees 150 patients a day might alleviate some suffering; however, the sick call patrol does not practice good medicine. Experience showed that medications provided were seldom, if ever, taken as directed. As most problems encountered were due to endemic communicable disease, treatment without follow-up leads to reinfection. As mentioned previously, the other main problem of poor hygiene and sanitation was also not properly addressed.

When asked whether they thought they had accomplished anything in the villages, responses, such as, "well, I probably saved a couple of people's lives. I don't know what side they're fighting on now. I do know there are some well trained Montagnard medics and Vietnamese medics there because of what we did,"[57] came from SF medics in 1965. A battalion surgeon of the Americal Division felt that the program fell short of its objectives, with little coordination between the battalion and the GVN and a lack of transportation for patients requiring hospitalization. There was a tendency of the GVN to allow the U.S. personnel to provide services rather than establishing their own system.[58] This experience paralleled that of the combat aspects of the war. Even as the U.S. experience in Vietnam lengthened and the program became better organized, the delivery of the care still took place in the same rudimentary settings in the villages and hamlets, most often school buildings. There was never an improvement in equipment with portable laboratory or X-ray facilities for MEDCAP II.

George F. Brockman, M.D., spent two months in Vietnam as a volunteer under the auspices of Project Vietnam. When he returned to the States, he reported that "the total medical accomplishment is little. But Vietnamese and American, civilian and medical, all unite in feeling that the offering of even a little medical care to a people who have never had any is winning the minds of the populace from the Communists with a weapon they cannot match."[59] His impression or "feeling" is unsupported by any data. General Westmoreland, in his July 1967 assessment report, noted that "the majority of the people in the rural areas appear apathetic towards the RD (Revolutionary Development, or civic action) effort. There has been no significant change in the people's attitude since their 'aspirations' are not being realized as rapidly as they would like, and the program is too limited in scope to have any significant effect on the majority of the citizens."[60]

The battalion surgeon of the 1st Battalion, 46th Infantry, 198th Infantry Brigade, Capt. David Allred, lucidly described the MEDCAP program. According to Allred, there was little coordination between the battalion and the GVN officials. Attempts to reach these officials were unsuccessful, and when reached, they were unwilling to provide information or services. Transportation to hospitals was unavailable when needed by patients seen on MEDCAP. It appeared to Allred that as long as services were provided by U.S. forces, there was no effort by the GVN to establish a permanent system to provide such services. Regardless of the number of patients treated, he regarded the MEDCAP program as ineffectual.[61] There was no basic change or improvement in the Vietnamese health care system.

Richard Austin served as deputy commander of the 44th Medical Brigade, therefore more on the command than the treatment end. In his opinion, the MEDCAP program "considerably helped" our relationships with the Vietnamese. He felt the best work was done in visiting the province hospitals because of the opportunity to consult with the Vietnamese doctors and actually help in caring for problem cases. In the villages, there were good public relations but not much medical benefit. He also recalled issues involving security, as when a doctor from the 93rd Evacuation Hospital found a claymore mine in the village square where he was to hold a MEDCAP.[62]

Dr. David Rioch, Director, Division of Neuropsychiatry, Walter

Reed Army Institute of Research (WRAIR), visited Vietnam in March and April 1964. He considered the civilian medical aid program as no more than a "traveling medicine show," part of the psychological warfare operations. As he phrased it, "Although such activities collect large numbers of villagers the procedure appears to confirm the peasant's belief in magic merely with the statement that Western magic is more powerful than local magic. Such a procedure may win an election, but in the long run it is truly dangerous and represents an inexcusable prostitution of medical facilities."[63]

Opinions like these were common. The hospital-based programs provided good medical care. They had the potential to improve the overall quality of Vietnamese medicine by teaching Vietnamese doctors and nurses. The village-based MEDCAP visits did help some individuals but forged no change in the basic medical care available to the rural population and were poorly suited to provide care to the seriously ill or long-term care for chronic diseases.

The quality of the medical care received varied considerably. Those who received care from a U.S. unit on a tactical mission received token care only, while those located in an area visited routinely by a MEDCAP team stationed in the locale for an extended time obtained far better care. Even the care of the latter group was frequently inadequate. The lack of diagnostic aids, such as laboratory or X-ray equipment, limited the ability of MEDCAP personnel to provide the type of medical care that they would otherwise be capable of providing.[64]

U.S. military hospitals admitted selected Vietnamese civilians for "high impact" surgical procedures. In this program, Vietnamese civilians, primarily children, with serious defects, deformities, and functional impairments were admitted for corrective surgery. These surgical procedures, performed on an elective basis, did not interfere with the primary mission of the hospital and, in fact, enhanced the morale and capabilities of army surgeons by providing humanitarian and professional opportunities between the demands of peak combat casualty load. The psychological impact on the inhabitants of the village to which the restored patient returned was tremendous.[65]

There is little discussion of the role of medical specialty care in MEDCAP activities. Reconstructive procedures for polio, leprosy, congenital deformities, and civilian war wounds were done at almost every hospital with an orthopedic surgeon whenever feasible. This was gratifying to both the patients and the surgeons. This aspect of civilian care was centered more in the MILPHAP than MEDCAP setting. Regrettably, these techniques were not shared with the Vietnamese physicians because of limited communications.[66]

Naval and army units participated in the programs. The naval medical corps officer Lt. H. E. Leventhal discovered that it was difficult to accomplish more than simple first aid measures. A significant language barrier existed. The people he saw had little knowledge or understanding of modern medicine and were reluctant to go to the hospital for admission or for testing. Further, after receiving medical care, the patients would return to the same environment with poor sanitary standards, which was not changed.[67] In other words, his experience paralleled that of the army doctors.

Another naval unit was lucky in patient selection, enabling it to gain the people's confidence. An old man with a tumor on the back of his head, which was a large benign cyst that had been present for many years, was taken to the hospital in Phu Bai and had the tumor removed in minor surgery. He was back in the village and cured in a very short time. Unknowingly, the navy doctors had treated the most sacred part of the body in Vietnamese belief. There was an increase in willingness to see the American doctors.[68]

The MILPHAP hospital assistance program received criticism as well. In his end-of-tour report, Ernest Feigenbaum complained,

"Over the past 13 months no significant regional GVN health representation has been available, thus obliging USAID regional health staffs to develop isolated projects with little relationship to Ministry of Health objectives." The lack of rapport with GVN health authorities impeded work to the extent that local cooperation beyond the basic treatment of hospitalized patients never materialized. This caused USAID to give first priority to curative medical projects with logistical systems patterned on military field hospital operations, therefore with no institution building potential. Health services for the "nonailing" majority tended to be neglected.[69]

The report was not fully accepted as it worked its way up the chain of command. The first endorser did not concur that the teams had failed to fulfill their stated objectives. He did note that "there has been great variation in the performance of these teams, usually equated to the military leadership qualities of their commanders who are often young two year service physicians." In other words, the plan was satisfactory, but the implementation was faulty. This is a clear example of the difference in positions taken by the command structure and the physicians involved. Despite this, the endorser did note the problems caused by the short rotations and the difficulties caused by the lack of overlap of the teams.[70]

Medical Corps Col. Raymond Bishop considered the MILPHAP program to be of considerable medical value, in contrast to the MEDCAP program. There were significant improvements in the capabilities of the provincial hospitals as soon as the teams were functional. The improved hospitals upgraded the entire civic action effort by providing a referral hospital for needy patients seen on MEDCAPs. The number of patients treated through MILPHAP and the attending publicity was not as great as with the MEDCAP teams, but the medical care received was "far superior."[71] By the time of the program termination on 30 June 1972, MACV headquarters felt it had been quite successful.

Construction projects for hospitals and dispensaries were carried out over a wide range of plans. Line units utilized their indigenous or normally supplied construction materials on a rather *ad hoc* basis to build some dispensaries and aid stations. Soldiers used spare lumber and tin for the roofs, working in their spare time. Other hospital projects were fully planned with architectural drawings and carried out by the Corps of Engineers and civilian contractors. Even these plans were frequently changed or derailed midway through the project. For example, the concept of building three special hospitals to care for Vietnamese civilians with war injuries was abandoned, and these patients were absorbed into the existing military hospital systems.

While there has been considerable discussion regarding the effect of the one-year tour, Col. John Sheedy, MC, highlighted another less frequently commented on problem. At about the sixth month of a tour, a "slight decline" in effectiveness occurred that is believed to be due to flagging enthusiasm as the project becomes routine or reaches a state of quiescence or semicompletion. A further decline occurred toward the end of the tour with a reluctance to begin new projects or correct errors in older projects. In a war zone with its attached dangers, there was a "natural inclination" to avoid taking chances.[72] Personnel, including physicians, became increasing reluctant to leave the base camps as the end of their tour approached. This "short-timers" syndrome (one was getting "short" as the number of days left in country decreased, especially to single digits) prevailed in both the combat and support forces.

Evaluation of any civic action or pacification program is difficult, with few objective measurements available. More could be inferred about the short-term impact of pacification than on the long-term effect in helping to create a sociopolitical environment in which future insurgency would not again flourish.[73] Further, even over the short term, it was hard to assess the relative extent to which observed changes in the countryside could be attributed to the pacification program as opposed to other factors. If this was true about the pacification program as a whole, then attributing benefit to one segment of the overall pacification program, in this instance medical care, would be even more problematic. Robert Komer, head of Civil Operations, Revolutionary Development Support (CORDS), concluded, "No real test of pacification's ultimate impact may ever be feasible."[74]

Komer did feel that pacification programs between 1967 and 1970 probably played a major role in reducing the effectiveness of the VC insurgency. He found the impact on the VC to be much greater than on the invading NVA units. This reasonable conclusion emphasizes the difference in the use of pacification and medical programs in a "traditional" war as opposed to a war of insurgency or a "limited" war. It also reinforces the problems of the United States in attempting to fight a limited war while the opposition was fighting a total or unlimited war.[75]

Col. Merle D. Thomas, the command surgeon in Vietnam, briefed a General Accounting Office team in country in October 1972. He noted the difficulty in separating the military and civilian medical capabilities in Vietnam, as they were intertwined and interrelated. According to Thomas, the close association between the military and civilian health sectors had a positive influence on the improvement of total health care in Vietnam. Foremost among the benefits of the joint programs was the training received by health professionals and nonprofessionals during their military service.[76] Much was contributed by U.S. medical efforts, but these efforts, at times, resulted in only temporary relief of a situation and contributed little to the long-term improvement in the health status of the Vietnamese.[77]

The real test of the MILPHAP achievements would have been to see if they continued after the withdrawal of U.S. forces and resulted in a significant change in health care delivery to the people. There is virtually no documentation regarding the programs in the 1973 (U.S. withdrawal) to April 1975 (fall of Saigon) period.

Unfortunately, after the fall of South Vietnam no studies of the impacts of the programs were possible.

When evaluating the medical impact of the various civilian medical programs, establishment of criteria is difficult but necessary. Tom Dooley was criticized for running hospitals that were not up to current standards of Western medicine. He responded, "In America doctors run 20th century hospitals. In Asia I run a 19th century hospital. Upon my departure the hospital may drop to the 18th century. This is fine, because previously the tribes in the high valleys lived, medically speaking, in the 15th century."[78] SF Lt. Col. Stanley Allison echoed these thoughts some thirty years later. "If you want to compare the medical care given to the care at Columbia Presbyterian Hospital in New York City, then it's fairly primitive." If the level began in the Dark Ages and is brought forward several hundred years, and it is better than anything they have ever had in their entire history, then it was worthwhile.[79]

Unquestionably, there were many instances of significant medical benefit from the MEDCAP program. Patients with infectious diseases were treated and cured, congenital deformities were corrected, reconstructive procedures were performed, and many Vietnamese had lifelong benefits from the program. Entire communities were immunized, achieving long-term medical benefits. Sanitation was improved, and programs were carried out to control plague and cholera. Some of the lessons taught in those programs might have persisted after the U.S. withdrawal.

Other episodes reflect less well on the U.S. attempts to win the hearts and minds through medical care. There were many single-visit MEDCAPs. There were too many road shows and traveling circuses with no adequate laboratory or radiological backup. Too often it was felt necessary to give something to everyone, whether there was any treatable disease present. Too often the medicines were given out on the basis that it was what was on hand and would not do any harm anyway. Too often interpreters were inadequate and dosages could not be explained, making the medications relatively worthless. Too often chronic diseases such as tuberculosis were treated symptomatically with cough syrup, or appropriate therapy was instituted only to be incomplete due to lack of follow-up. If the medical benefits of the program were limited, perhaps the deficiencies were offset by the benefits to U.S. aims of offering civilians medical assistance. These policy considerations will be examined in the next chapter.

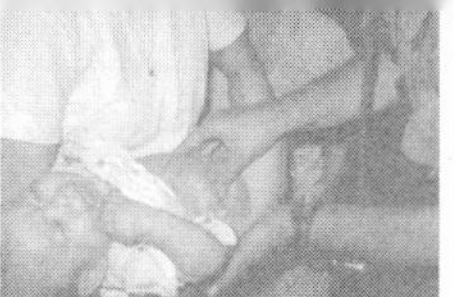

Six
Evaluation of the Programs as a Policy Tool

There is an old adage that if you give a man a fish, he has a meal to eat; but if you teach him to fish, he can feed himself for life. Trite but true. Clearly, caring for the sick and injured is a good thing, but does it have lasting benefit? It is far less dramatic to build a training program that can take years to deliver a benefit, even though a training program has the potential to change society and be of long-lasting benefit. There may well be less publicity associated with a training program as well as less glory and gratitude associated with it. Discussion of the various programs for delivery of health care to civilians constitutes a "micro" view. The "macro" questions are (1) whether medicine can be a significant instrument of policy and (2) if so, whether medicine was used in an effective manner during the Vietnam conflict.

In Chapter 5, it is notable that none of the physicians or other health providers considered the policy questions when evaluating the programs. They were concerned about the quality of medicine being provided to the people and distressed by their perceived inability to render care in what they thought was an acceptable manner. They were not involved in the discussions or decisions as to whether to institute the programs, and, in fact, much of their participation was significantly less voluntary than the command structure suggested. Unit commanders were tasked with carrying out civic action programs, and the medical personnel were part of that program. The doctor was not asked whether he wished to MEDCAP, he was told to do so.

In contrast to the physicians, the command structure indicated little or no interest in the quality of medical care provided. It was important to participate in the program, and the more patients seen, the more medicines and medical supplies distributed, the better the program was functioning to aid the war effort. This was consistent with the Secretary of Defense Robert S. McNamara's system of evaluating the war effort by measuring the body count or the amount of munitions and bombs expended. Higher numbers were equated with progress and evidence of winning the war. Further, it was necessary for each unit commander to surpass his predecessor in all quantifiable tasks to maximize his own OER.

MAAG recognized that MEDCAP was not an example of the highest quality of medical service that the United States could offer the world.[1] MEDCAP was never intended to be a purely medical effort, but primarily intended as psychological aid to combating VC infiltration. The author of the MAAG study thought it was possible that those opposed to the program never understood its underlying principles or stimulus. I would maintain from personal experience that if that is correct, it is in great part because the command structure never discussed or explained this to those actively engaged in carrying out the program. Objections to MEDCAPing were met with orders to continue participating in the program, rather than any discussion of the motives underlying it. The program was not as purely voluntary as the American public was led to believe. This in no way is at odds with many nurses, doctors, and medics who found participation in civic action programs the most rewarding part of their tour in Vietnam.

MAAG felt that caring for civilians could be an opening wedge to create contact with the people of Vietnam, allowing other activities in the future. The VC could oppose improvements in structures such as roads and fortifications. Buildings, such as schools or dispensaries, or structures, such as roads or bridges, could be and often were destroyed by the VC to show the inability of the GVN to have a lasting effect.[2] The VC were less likely to try to bar medical people because they helped the people in a manner that the people desired.

The official MACV position was that MEDCAP played an important role in the overall civic action program in Vietnam. U.S. field advisors reported that "no other civic action project has had a more immoderate and dramatic effect than has MEDCAP." Aside from the medical aspects of the program, it was considered to be an "extremely valuable tool in the area of psychological operations." The appearance of medical personnel in rural areas served as evidence of interest in the welfare of the people. Treatment of the rural people "contributed to their better understanding of the American soldiers and their presence in Vietnam."[3] The Medical Service Report of the 2nd Battalion, 22nd Infantry described the recipients of the MEDCAP care as "always enthusiastic in their gratitude."[4] An additional benefit was that MEDCAP served to assemble many people who could then be given GVN "information."[5]

While dramatic successful procedures clearly had the potential to win over the populace, medical success was not always necessary for the programs to have a positive impact. The obvious distress manifested by two U.S. Navy surgeons on the death of a Buddhist girl after a four-hour fight to save her life was observed by a suspicious Buddhist bonze (or monk) at Bao Loc in Lam Dong Province in the Central Highlands. The monk, Thay Thanh, and an associate, Thay Quang, who had been a leader of anti-American student riots in 1966 in Hué, became convinced that the Americans were "well-motivated" and supported their efforts.[6]

USARV Surgeon Spurgeon Neel (who served tours as MACV

Surgeon in 1965 and USARV Surgeon in 1969) felt that participation in humanitarian programs "provided U.S. medical personnel gainful and rewarding activity during lulls between peak military medical support requirements. This, in turn, contributed to the high morale of committed U.S. 'medics.'"[7] This was important as doctors could basically not be given nonmedical duties, according to regulation. This was especially true in a war zone, where, for example, one would not want a doctor to serve as officer-of-the-day and have the potential to be in a position to command troops.

Gen. William C. Westmoreland considered doctors and nurses, even in uniform, as "civilian specialists."[8] He further observed that medical personnel "are discontent, even feel misused, when they are not occupied with their specialty."[9] He felt doctors "were the biggest bunch of letter writers in the world."[10] Westmoreland felt the only thing doctors and nurses knew how to do wholesomely was take care of sick people; if they weren't taking care of our own casualties, he wanted them busy doing the thing they did best, taking care of other sick people. Lt. Col. Gene Aaby worked in the office of the USARV Surgeon. He commented that "surgeons like to work." They are unhappy if they are not busy, and he received complaints from the surgeons assigned to the divisions who were not busy professionally.[11] Neel described the effort to keep the doctors busy as a "conscious decision."[12] This unpublicized reasoning was not acknowledged as a reason to embark on these programs during the conflict.

The typical situation in which U.S. military medical units are deployed in counterinsurgency situations is one of considerable excess medical capacity. This is reasonable and necessary so that when significant numbers of casualties occur, there will be adequate personnel available to care for them. It is the same reason that there should always be empty beds in the hospital units. The medical commander must keep his staff busy to preserve their morale and technical competence and keep them from being siphoned off on other details. This applies to the enlisted technicians and specialists, rather than to the physicians. The enlisted personnel could be given other duties such as KP, guard duty, etc., when not occupied with those tasks involved with medical care. If this occurred frequently enough, some of the enlisted personnel could effectively be lost to the medical section. Also, when the need arose for their medical abilities they might be committed to other duties and unable to participate in the medical effort.

Additional pressure toward MEDCAP operations came from the ever-present need to maintain good public relations in the United States. According to Medical Corps Col. James Kirkpatrick, nonviolent activities that seem to contribute to the well-being of the host country are much more presentable in the mass media than are combat operations.[13] There was a ready audience in the hometown newspapers for stories about MEDCAP and especially pertaining to the care of children.

In limited warfare situations, the Army Medical Department (AMEDD) civic action operations potential is greatest when applied in a preinsurgency phase. Once insurgency has begun, AMEDD's resources must be devoted to the conventional combat support and related civil affairs tasks. This diverts AMEDD resources away from activities that have permanent effects on the stability of the host nation.[14] In this regard, it is important to recognize the true nature of the conflict, i.e., whether it is truly a "limited war."

An Office of the Surgeon General study noted that the far-flung U.S. Army Medical support system requires the AMEDD to make extensive use of paramedical personnel. These personnel are, for the most part, created from "medically untrained civilians." An identical training requirement lies at or near the heart of a successful medical program in the countries the United States assists.[15] The army organization and delivery of medical services is at a level that has a potential to make a contribution to solving the health problems in underdeveloped nations. The Surgeon General's office considered that the AMEDD has a greater potential to make a contribution to solving the health problems of these nations than the civilian sector.[16] The study does not address the question of doing so by direct delivery of health care as opposed to training programs for indigenous health workers.

Military medicine, even in its most altruistic guise, is also an instrument to be used during low-intensity conflicts (as opposed to total war).[17] The strongest pressure for medical civic action has come from the humanitarian impulses of the medical people themselves. A mixture of boredom and a commendable desire to help the citizens of the host country led many physicians, nurses, and other medical personnel to seek opportunities to offer their services.[18] This altruistic tendency coincided with the wishes of the command structure at the highest levels for participation in the programs. This altruistic inclination is in no way a contradiction to resistance to the way the program was conducted, often on a nonvolunteer basis over the objections of the physicians. This pressure from above to participate in medical civic action came from higher headquarters, the Department of the Army and the Office of the Secretary of Defense. Documents show interest from "the highest level," that is, the president of the United States, in these programs.[19]

It would appear that doing "good" should not be open to debate and criticism. When asked about the effectiveness of medical aid in winning the hearts and minds of the Vietnamese, USARV Surgeon Maj. Gen. Spurgeon Neel pointed out that the Vietnamese could not understand why we (the U.S. military) were doing this, as no one had ever done anything for them before. Further, that "there was the feeling on the military side that 'good works' was a bonus."[20]

Many officers and medics indicated that helping the civilians was the most gratifying experience they had during the war. Many doctors developed a "missionary spirit."[21] Neel stated that "One hare lip [cleft lip] repair is worth a thousand bags of cement in winning the hearts and minds of the people."[22] The psychological impact on the inhabitants of the village to which a restored patient was returned was tremendous. In 1963, MAAG concluded, "It appeared militarily reasonable to use the army medical effort as part of an overall program of Military Civic Action."[23] The Army Medical Service was felt to make a major contribution toward winning the "other war" in Vietnam.[24]

General Westmoreland felt that the "nation building" aspects of U.S. civic action programs failed to receive the attention that was deserved, and Edward Glick noted the problems in evaluating the programs without satisfactory objective criteria.[25] When he assumed MACV command in 1964, Westmoreland felt that the campaign would be won at the "province, district, village and hamlet levels where the battle is being waged for the hearts and minds of the people."[26] His opinion in this regard would change after the battle of Ia Drang in 1965 when he adopted a strategy of seeking main force confrontations and a policy of attrition. Further, by 1967, he was voicing doubts about the effectiveness of the programs, stating that "the majority of the people in the rural areas appear apathetic toward the RD [Revolutionary Development or civic action program] effort. There has been no significant change in the people's attitude since their 'aspirations' are not being realized as rapidly as they would like, and the program is too limited in scope to have any significant effect on the majority of the citizens."[27]

Both medical and line units began various civic action projects a soon as they landed in Vietnam. The 85th Evacuation Hospital medical civic action activities began shortly after the unit arrived "in country." Recognition of the acute need existing for even rudimentary medical care in the civilian population provided the initial motivation for the program. Reconstructive procedures among the children received special emphasis, especially to correct congenital deformities.

The 85th Evacuation Hospital newsletter concluded that it was an obligation of our medical heritage to treat the sick, wherever they were found, and that medicine could offer one of the brightest hopes for Vietnam.[28] Hospital personnel became aware that the gains in goodwill were realized among the indigenous civilians for a fraction of the cost of other expenditures directed to other facets of U.S. military presence in the country. In considering medical strategy, Col. Edwin Carns (MC, retired) noted that many feel that military medicine is one of the most effective and least controversial means of employing military assets in a low-intensity conflict situation.[29]

Not all agree with using military medical personnel for other than treating the wounded. Barry S. Levy and Victor W. Sidel in *War and Public Health* clearly imply that any use of medical care to advance a war effort is immoral and wrong. They cite the trial of Howard Levy, an army dermatologist who refused an order to train SF aidmen with the argument that the "political use of medicine by the Special Forces jeopardized the entire tradition of the noncombatant status of medicine." Even Col. James Kirkpatrick, writing in support of the use of military medicine in low-intensity conflicts, refers to the Geneva Convention that states medical care in war must be provided in a nondiscriminatory and noncoercive fashion.[30] There is, however, no requirement that medical care be provided to civilians.

The previously mentioned Howard Levy considered that doctors were not apolitical, but rather promoted the agenda of their commanders while using their abilities to treat civilians. Up until the Vietnam conflict, he considered that physicians served a supportive role for the troops, but in Vietnam, the physicians assumed a direct political role. He traced this back to Gen. Leonard Wood, who in the Philippines consciously used public health measures to pacify insurgent ethnic groups. To Levy, medicine had become an arm of American foreign policy.[31] His public dissent and failure to carry out lawful orders led to his court-martial.

Richard A. Falk, a physician and critic of the war who ultimately received a general discharge from the military for anti-war activities with four-and-a-half years of obligation remaining, did work in civic action while serving in Vietnam. He noted "modest" success in medical care in rural villages, public health and immunization programs, and evacuation of those requiring hospitalization or surgery. "Some necessary surgery was done, many acute illnesses benefited from antibiotic therapy, and a start was made on long-term treatment of tuberculosis cases."

Falk felt unable to treat adequately "any but the most superficial problems." He noted that the official policy of dispensing only a two-day supply of medications to prevent excesses falling into the hand of the VC, coupled with the irregularity of visits to any village prevented adequate medical treatment. He described the result as "a parody of medical care unsatisfying to both patients and physicians, most of whom feel quite cynical about their role in this charade." The exercise did, however, "produce multitudes of pictures for home consumption of Americans looking concerned about Vietnamese." Falk concluded that physicians should not agree to participate in the civilian care programs or in the war in any manner.[32] He therefore objected to the use of military medicine to aid the civilians on both policy and medical grounds.

Aside from the humanitarian reasons for the various civilian medical aid programs, Spurgeon Neel thought that medical services were properly used for political gains. MEDCAP was a tactical employment of medical capability to "try and influence the people we were there trying to help."[33] He believed the programs had a major impact on the psychological warfare campaign.[34] Neel also felt that another reason for the programs was that they improved the image of the United States.[35]

The ultimate success of any civic action program depends on the permanence of local improvements and the consequent improvement in rapport between the national government and the local population.[36] There are two major points in that sentence: (1) the concept of permanence and (2) the rapport to be established between the local population and the national government. This is quite different from establishing a rapport between U.S. military forces and the local population, which is, of course, also laudable and useful but has entirely different policy implications.

Nonrecurrent civic action can be worse than no civic action at all.[37] A program that leaves some in a village or neighborhood untreated can create hard feelings. Their ill will might exceed the goodwill of those who were treated.[38] Ending programs can be difficult, and raising the expectations of the population and then dashing them might be counterproductive. This problem was encountered during and after the Tet 1968 battles, when civic action and rural development teams and their security forces were withdrawn from the countryside to fight in the cities. It enabled the enemy to show that it was a more permanent force than was the government or the foreign (U.S.) forces.

For many years, the Providence Orphanage in Can Tho, in the Mekong Delta, received help from the American GIs and American Navy doctors. The doctors received generous gifts from the Pennsylvania Academy of General Practice; clothing from the Messiah Lutheran Church in Whitemash, Pennsylvania; and drug samples from both Merck, Sharpe, and Dome and Smith, Kline, and French manufacturers. Gerber Baby Foods sent baby food and formula; Johnson & Johnson sent baby care products. According to Sister Eugenia, the orphanage received only 100,000 piasters a month from the GVN, while their expenses came to three times that, 300,000 piasters (in the late 1960s and early 1970s, the official exchange rate was roughly 118 piasters to the U.S. dollar). The U.S. Navy gave the orphanage the additional funds, plus boxes of clothing and medications, in addition to the services of navy doctors. As the unit stand-down from Vietnam was underway in 1972, the doctors immunized the children. They felt this was something that would last after the U.S. withdrawal. Both the doctors and the sisters worried, not knowing where the necessary help for the orphanage would come from after the U.S. units left the country.[39]

The traditional medical civic action program is a classic example of impatience mixed with goodwill. The traditional MEDCAP might be counterproductive to the overall goal of creating confidence in the local government. It might foster a false impression about the local government's ability and desire to meet the population's needs by building expectations that cannot be met after the U.S. personnel departure.[40] It is important to constantly reiterate that the goal of the programs must be to build support for the local government that the United States is backing, not to gain support and friendship for U.S. military forces abroad.

Rather than emphasizing the overall improvement in the health of the population, production factors, such as number of patients seen, number of teeth extracted, and number of vaccinations given received the most attention. In general, there was "too much worry about figure totals and not enough about the quality of treatment."[41] This method of evaluation was consistent with the manner in which Secretary of Defense Robert McNamara conducted the war: his road to success lay in his specialty, statistical control.[42] USAID recognized that statistical measure of the supplies used did not adequately evaluate the programs, but an evaluation of the accomplishments in improvement of the health environment within Vietnam was needed.[43]

While one person occupied both the position of commander, USARV, and commander, MACV, the coordination of the program was through the MACV surgeon and not the army (USARV) surgeon. The payment for the supplies came through MACV, not through USARV or the III MAF. If a battalion surgeon held sick call in the morning, his supplies came through USARV as that was the logistical side, and his medical reports went to USARV. If the same doctor went into the village in the afternoon, his supplies and reporting were through MACV, as that was a tactical operation.

Several factors made it virtually impossible to determine

accurately the amount of funds expended in Vietnam for civilian medical care. Many of the programs were conducted informally or on an ad hoc basis, especially during the early years of U.S. involvement. Supplies and funds for civilian medical care were not separated from those used in routine care of military personnel and their dependents, allies, etc. It would have been rather onerous for battalion size units to try to keep the supplies separate and was not feasible. Small units such as SF A teams relied on scrounging and bartered to obtain many supplies, none of which was recorded. Battalion medical units sometimes traded medical supplies with SF medics for souvenirs such as small arms and captured weapons. I can personally attest to this occurring, as I observed it on more than a few occasions. Charitable organizations within the United States contributed medical supplies, clothing, and money, especially for the support of orphanages. Many of these gifts were sent directly to soldiers, sailors, and airmen for distribution because they had solicited them from their hometowns. They were never formally recorded.

Furthermore, accurate accounting is difficult due to the plethora of organizations involved in the different programs. In some cases, the funding was hidden within other appropriations, either intentionally or unintentionally. Military units often used excess medical supplies for MEDCAP-type programs. Some programs were conducted by agencies, such as the CIA, whose budgets were never fully disclosed (and whose papers have not yet been opened for study). Other civic action and medical care programs were simply part of the regular tasks of the units, such as engineering units, and not specifically separated out of the budget. For example, engineering units might build a dispensary in off-duty hours with leftover construction materials. This activity would be reported as an accomplished civic action task but would never show up on any budget or ledger sheet. In some instances, funding for medical programs was a part of civic action or pacification allocations but not specifically separated out as a distinct budgetary line item. Medical care to civilians rendered

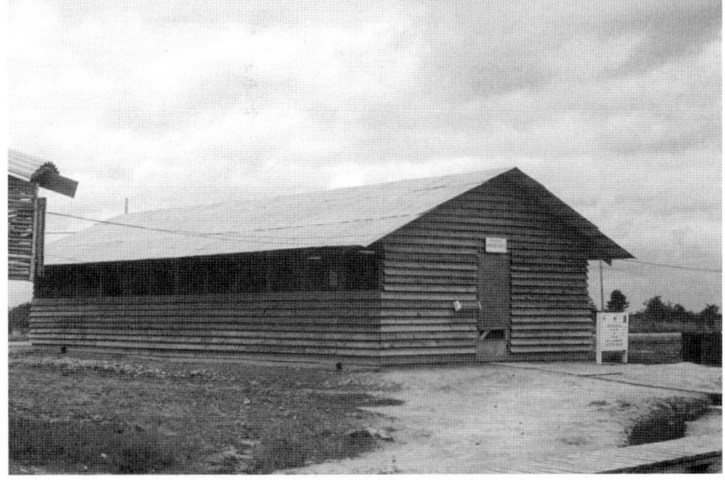

The author's 588th Engineer Battalion (C) (A) aid station at Tay Ninh Base Camp.

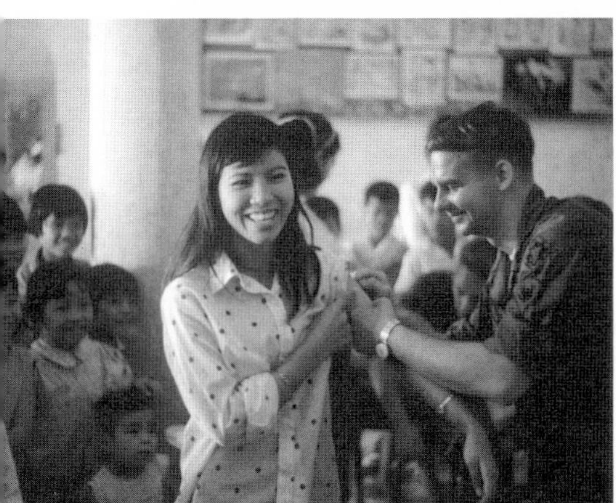

The 588th Engineer Battalion aid station's interpreter, Vi Hui, receives a fake shot to show the children it would not hurt.

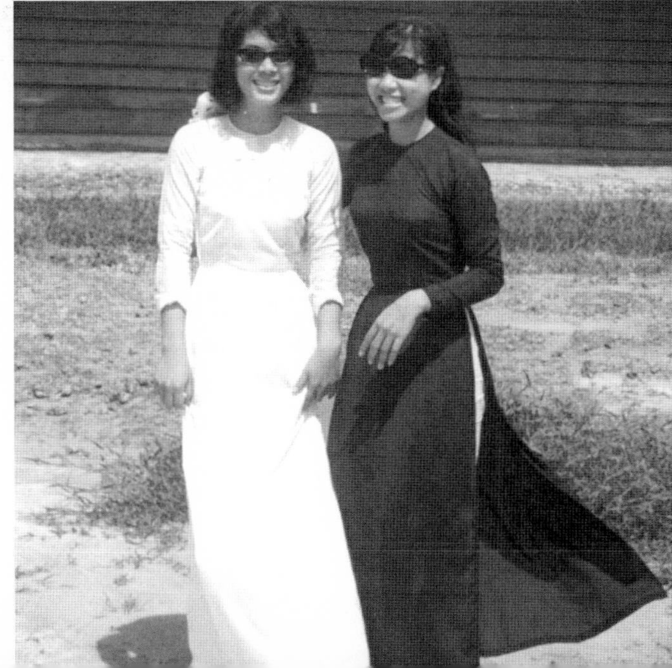

Interpreter Vi Hui (right) and her sister, Trung Vi, in *ao dai,* the traditional Vietnamese dress. Although they were trained as nurses, they made more money working as interpreters for the U.S. Army.

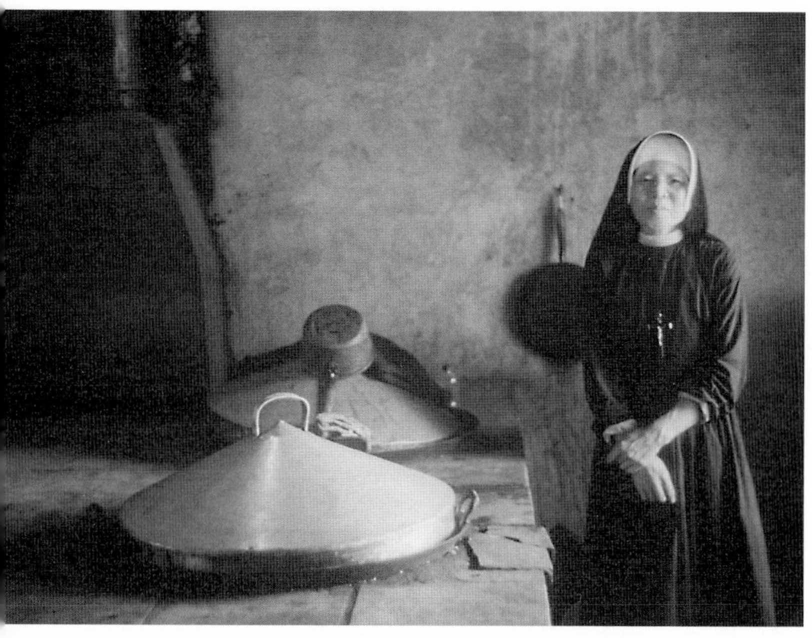

In these two woks this nun cooked all the meals for the children at the Cau Dai Orphanage in Tay Ninh.

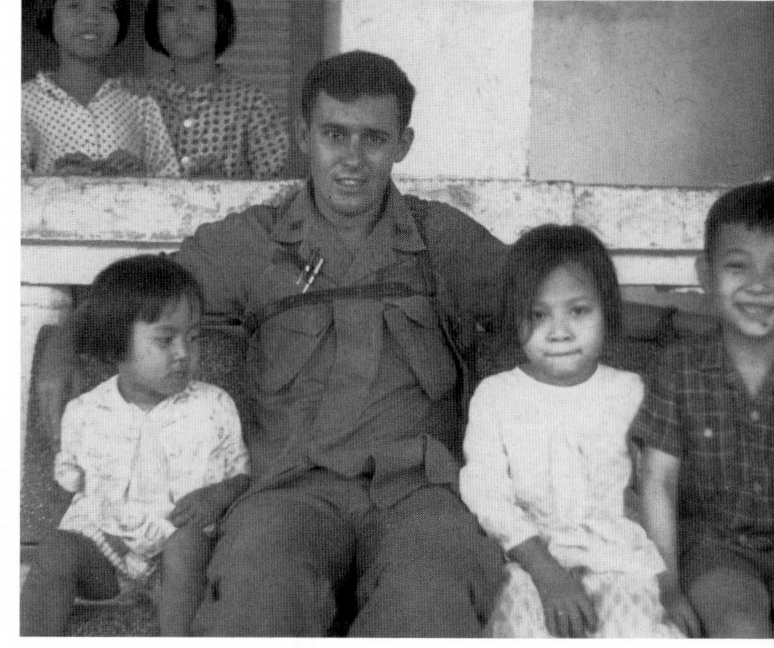

The author with some of the children at the Cau Dai Orphanage.

Spc. 5 Bailey giving an immunization to an infant.

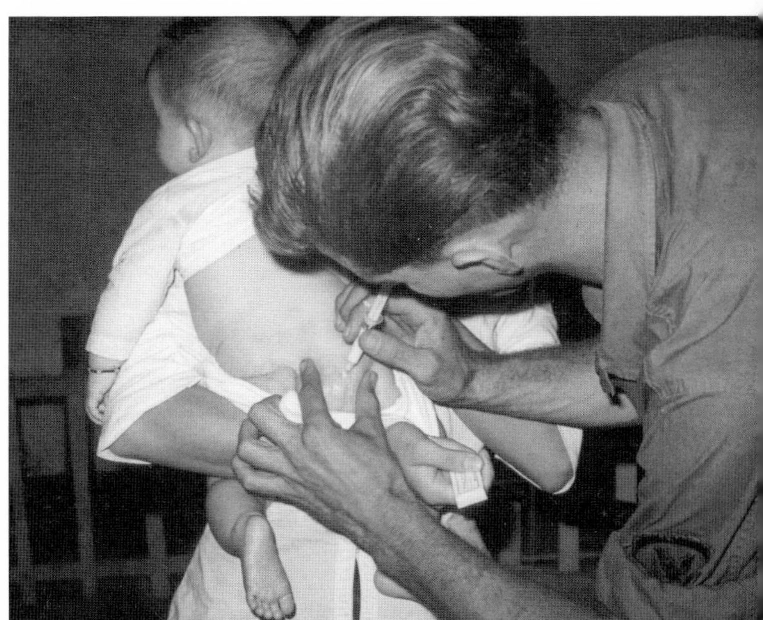

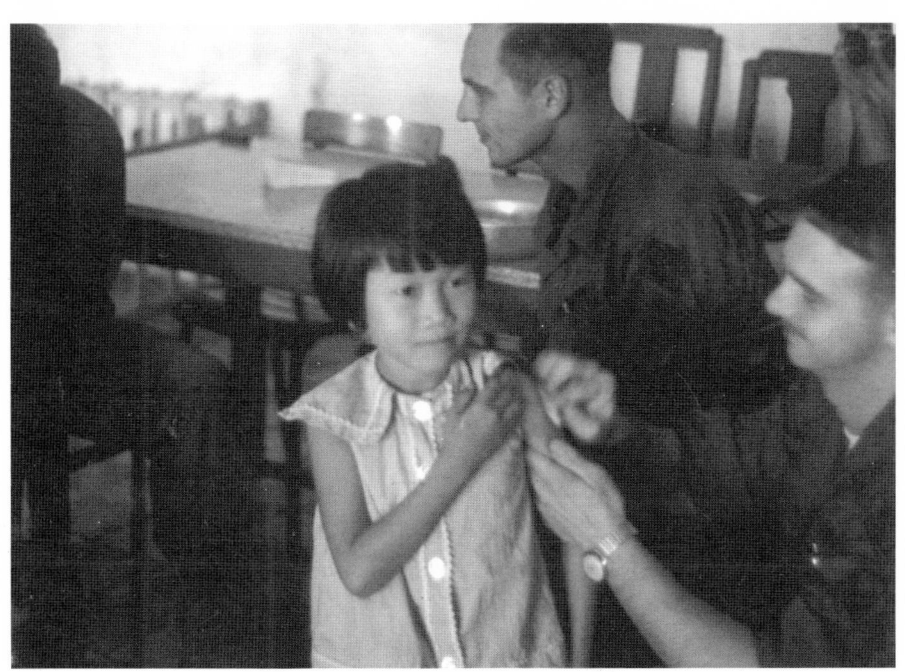

Spc. 4 Chandler giving an immunization to an older child.

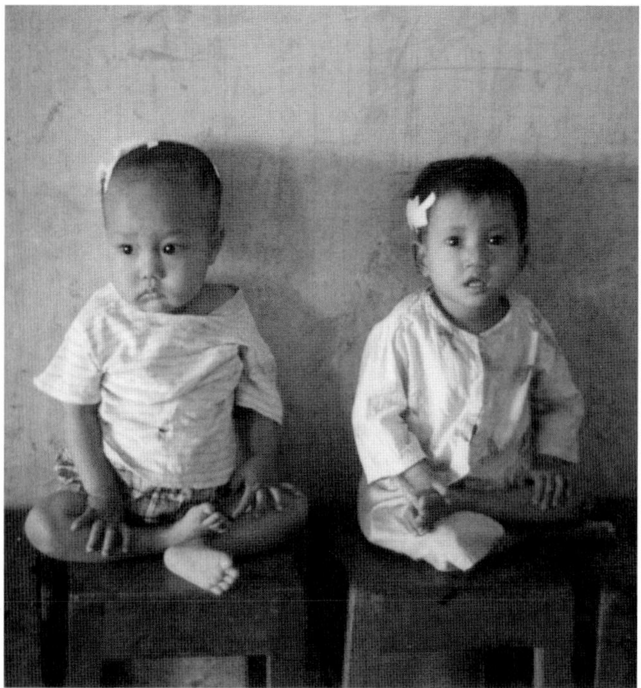

Two children from the orphanage with scalp skin infections.

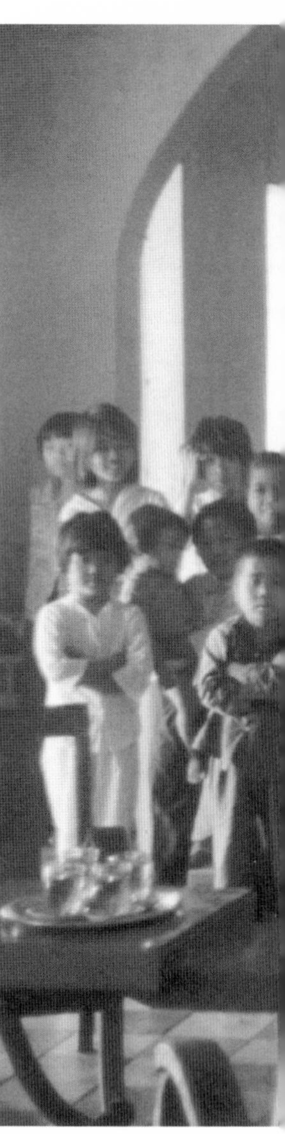

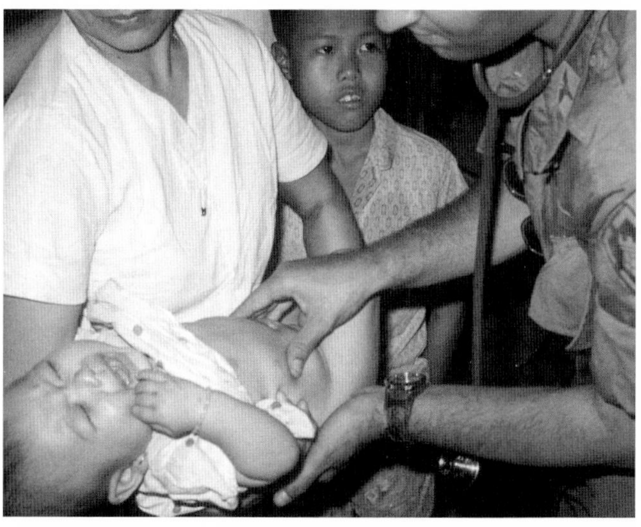

The author examining an infant in the orphanage.

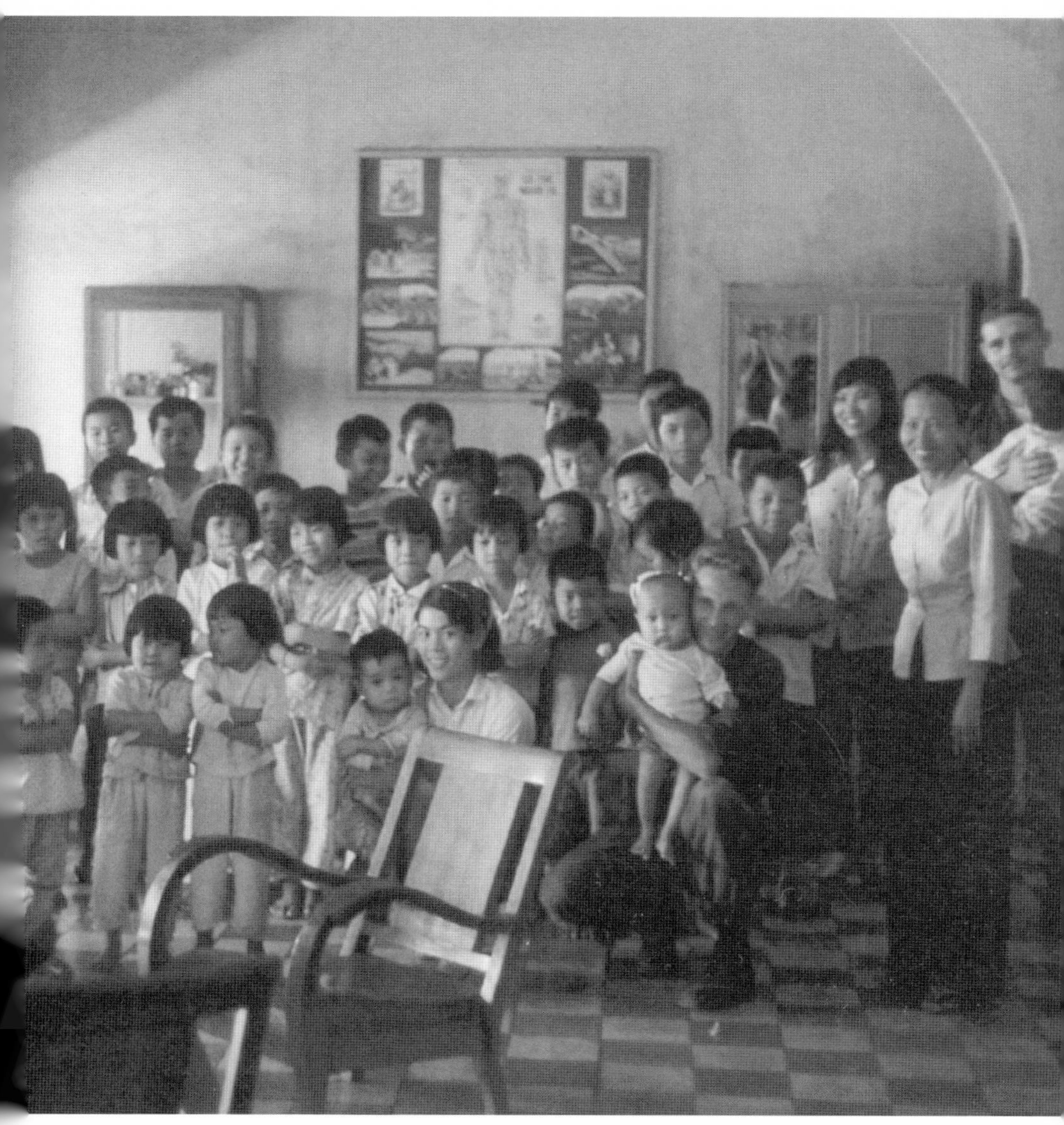

After the author and his team finished examining and treating the children at the orphanage, the children serenaded them.

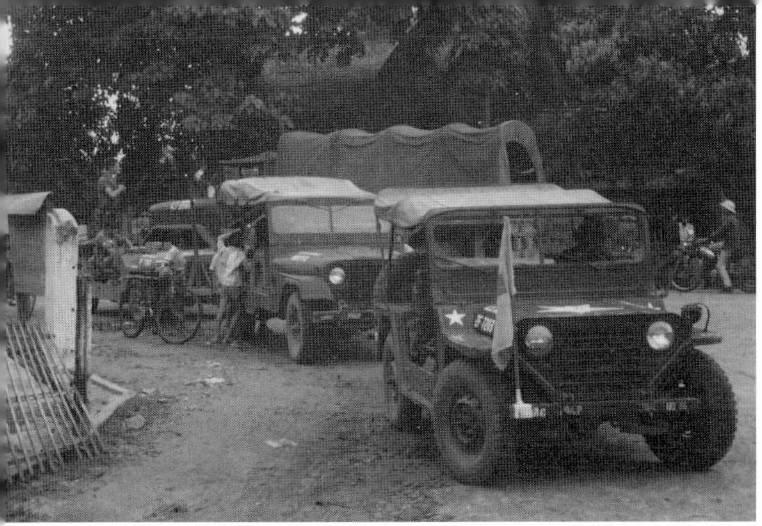

The 588th Engineer Battalion aid station's MEDCAP convoy at Sui Da, near Tay Ninh in III Corps.

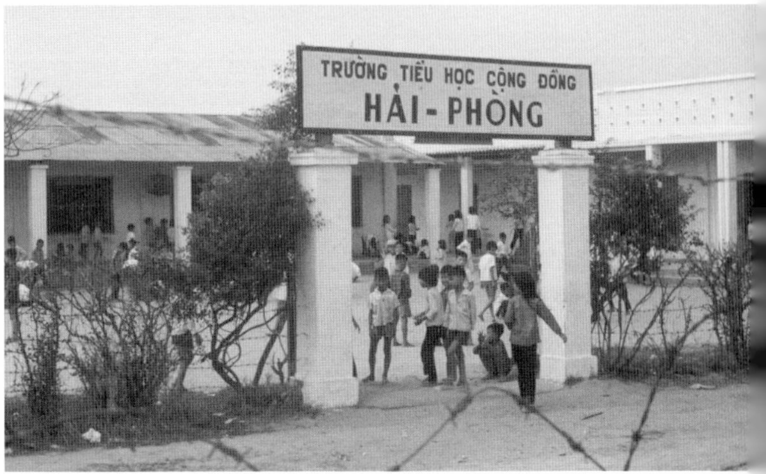

The author also held MEDCAP at this school in Bien Hoa.

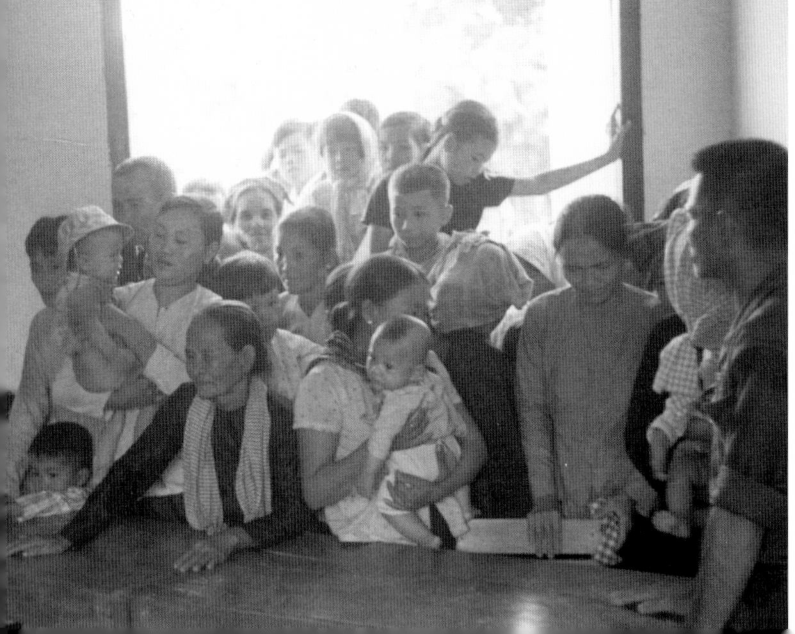

Civilians crowd into the waiting area for MEDCAP aid.

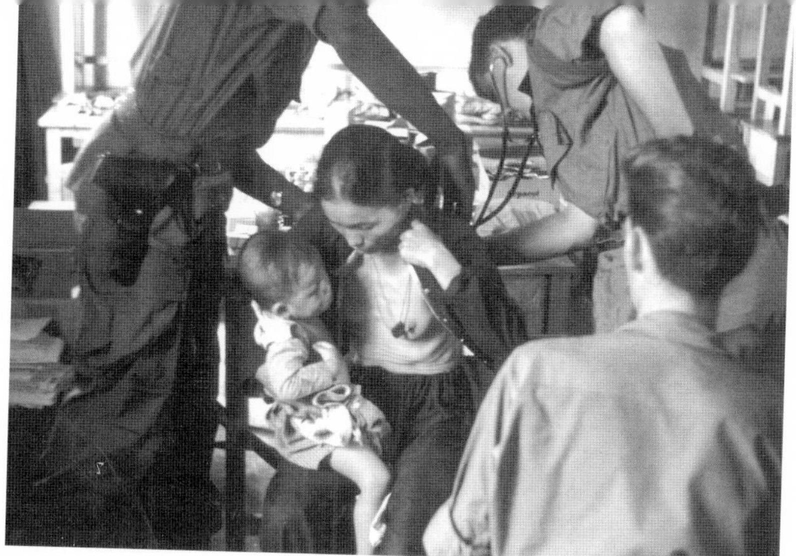

Medics examine a woman while she feeds her infant.

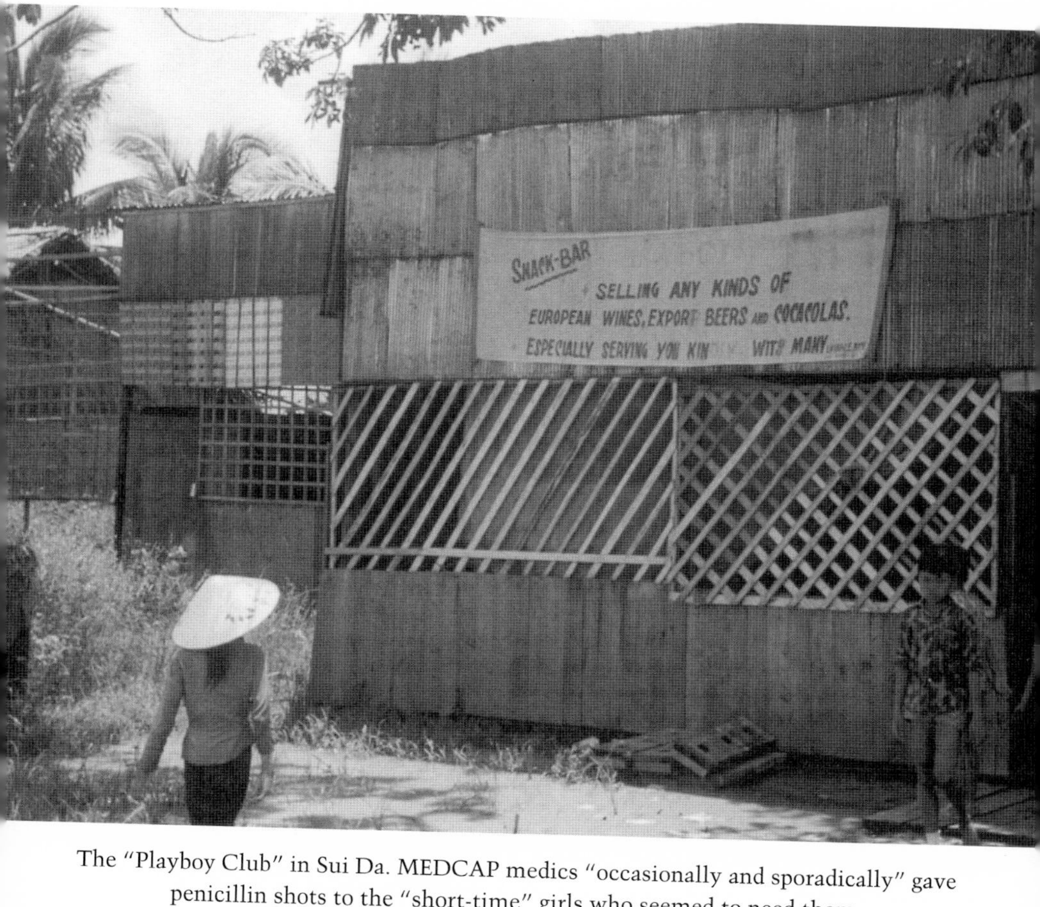

The "Playboy Club" in Sui Da. MEDCAP medics "occasionally and sporadically" gave penicillin shots to the "short-time" girls who seemed to need them. There were no lab facilities on MEDCAP.

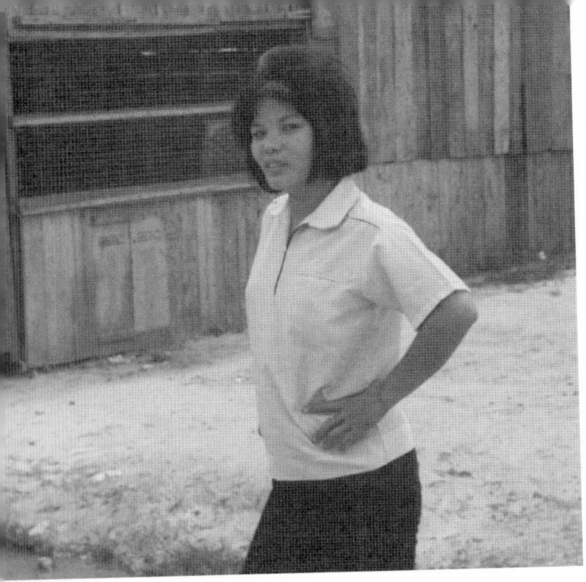

One of the "short-time" girls from the "Playboy Club." She showed symptoms typical of gonorrhea, for which she was treated, but the MEDCAP team had no laboratory documentation to support the diagnosis.

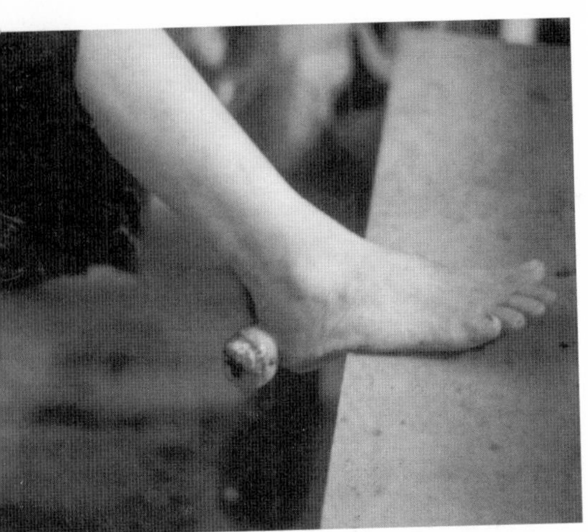

A tumor on the heel of a woman seen on MEDCAP at Sui Da. The patient was referred to the provincial hospital for treatment, as the team was not equipped to handle her case, but there was no way to know if she ever went there.

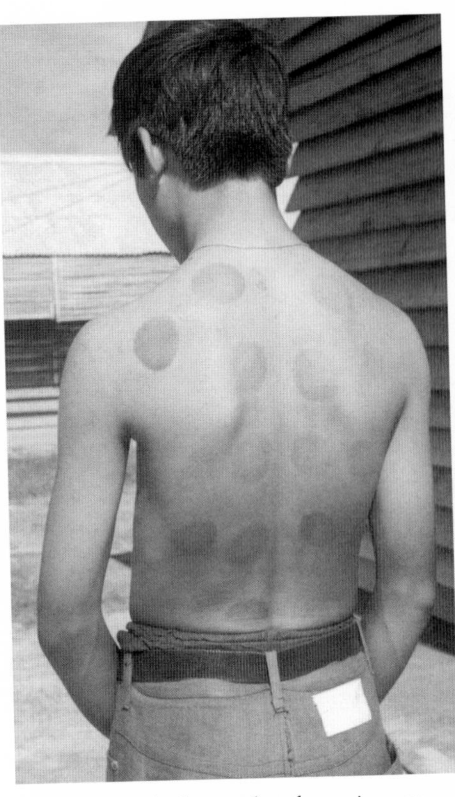

A boy with the marks of cupping, an ancient folk treatment practiced in many societies. Very few young men of working or military age were seen on MEDCAPs.

during tactical maneuvers was often unreported or underreported. Supplies utilized for these treatments came from those carried on the maneuver, not from the MEDCAP supply system. Lastly, at the time of U.S. withdrawal from Vietnam, a great deal of materials and numerous buildings were turned over to the Vietnamese. It is impossible to determine how much of this was medical in nature.

Any figure for the total expenditures for civilian medical aid is an approximation. Totaling expenditures listed by USAID, MAAG, MACV, Department of Army (DA), and DOD amounts to at least $185,000,000, and adding FWMAF funds for civilian health care brings the total to over $350,000,000 for the period of 1963 to 1973.[44] This includes funds expended for CWCP hospital construction, MILPHAP, MEDCAP, and PHAP. The significance of the figure is in the order of magnitude, rather than the specific amount. This figure is not great if compared to expenditures for munitions and bombs, but it is clearly not insignificant. It raises the question as to whether suitable value was obtained from this expenditure to make it worthwhile as an instrument of policy.

The many organizations involved in medical care for civilians also has other implications. There were the various U.S. governmental branches and services, the FWMAF (many of which agreed to provide help to civilians rather than fighting men), various charities like faith-based groups and churches, and other nondenominational charitable groups, such as CARE and Project HOPE, what would now be lumped under the general category of NGOs. Each of these organizations believed that it would benefit from providing medical care. As long as several organizations were providing medical care for civilians, there was no *one* individual or organization in control of these programs or responsible for their success or failure.

Numerous other smaller volunteer groups participated in the relief efforts. Dr. Carl E. Bartecchi, who served as a medical corps officer in Vietnam from October 1965 to October 1966, reported the support for the Soc Trang Orphanage from World Medical

Relief.[45] This organization, based in Detroit, began in 1953 to help the children of Korea after that war. One of the corpsmen working with Bartecchi was from Detroit and his appeal for clothing and medications in the *Detroit Free Press* resulted in support of their orphanage in the Mekong Delta. Another group was Operation Helping Hand, based in Hawaii, the home of the 25th Infantry Division. It provided 442 tons of materials over one six-month period for orphanage support.[46]

Graft, corruption, thievery, and even diversion of supplies to the enemy all occurred. It is impossible to determine the amounts.[47] SF units reported capturing VC with American medicines. Items were sold on the streets through the black market. VC and their dependents were treated during MEDCAP sick calls, hospitalized under the CWCP, and probably operated on in U.S. military facilities. They were even trained as medics by units conducting local on-the-job training programs. Retrospective reconstruction of accurate figures in this regard remains impossible.

Some special dangers are associated with the flow of civic action support from one country to another. Theoretically, such help is supposed to be from the foreign army to the host army and then from the host army to that country's civilians. Again, the aim of these programs is to build support for the government of the host country, not to engender warm feelings toward the U.S. military. There was ongoing concern with putting the Vietnamese in the forefront of the programs. As Brig. Gen. James Collins Jr. stated, "Civic action must start at the Rice Roots level. We must not get in a position where we overwhelm or compete with the GVN. We are in support of GVN efforts and operate within the GVN program. We are trying to build up the Government of Vietnam, not the U.S. You must, in civic action projects, keep the proper GVN authority in the foreground and the limelight."[48] In this regard in the medical arena, it was necessary to restrict medical aid to civilians to those areas where civilian medical resources were most lacking to avoid undermining the prestige and function of the civilian health workers in the area.[49]

In practice, however, it often turns out the foreign army frequently serves the local civilians directly. This certainly was true with MEDCAP II, which was what the program was intended to do. The villagers then are grateful to the foreign army, not their own army. It can even result in feelings that the foreign army not only fights but also cares about the civilians and helps them more than their own army.[50] One Vietnamese peasant put it into these chilling words: "Why are the American soldiers so good to us while our own government and soldiers do nothing for us?"[51] Another problem arose when Vietnamese physicians went out with the MEDCAP team. The population seemed to feel that American medicine and medical personnel were better than the Vietnamese ones and to prefer to be treated by the American doctors.[52] This clearly was not winning support for the Vietnamese government.

When speaking of the role of the soldiers in all civic action programs, General Westmoreland pointed out that in many parts of the country the soldier was often the only, or at least the primary, representative of the government in the people's eyes. The soldier must, therefore, convince the people that the government has their best interests at heart. No amount of words or propaganda will convince the people if the actions and conduct of the soldiers demonstrate otherwise.[53]

ARVN civic action efforts were spotty. ARVN troops appeared unwilling to provide all-out support for civic action efforts. This was considered, in part, because the ARVN soldier and his family usually had living conditions inferior to those of the population he was called on to assist.[54] These conditions also created situations where the ARVN appropriated rice and other food from the peasants and committed such crimes as rape. These activities were not permitted with VC cadres or by the NVA. (This is not to suggest that the VC and NVA were innocent of atrocities, but the routine conduct of their soldiers was intended to win over the peasantry, not alienate them.)

General Westmoreland felt that among the many civic action projects undertaken in Vietnam, "perhaps none had a more immediate and dramatic effect that the Medical Civic Action Program."[55] The MACV Surgeon recognized early on that the medical aid must appear to come from the central government, either a Vietnamese civilian or an ARVN soldier. If the U.S. or FWMAF medic was identified as the giver, it hurt the psychological war effort as it made the GVN representative appear to be subservient. Every effort had to be made to make the U.S. advisor or medical personnel stand in the background. "If the program is to accomplish its purpose of selling the GVN, the MEDCAP medic must enhance the work of the GVN representative and always make it look like he is in charge."[56] The U.S. medical advisor should stand in the background teaching and advising, "while the RVN medical personnel take the credit for improving the health of the rural population."[57] This was difficult for the U.S. personnel, as frequently they could accomplish the treatment or provide the care more rapidly and effectively by themselves. To be successful, the work had to be done so as to not draw so much attention to the U.S. forces that the gratitude and loyalty of the people flows to the United States rather than the host government. That was the most difficult part of the entire effort.[58] It certainly was not the way the MEDCAP II program developed with U.S. units providing direct care to the people. Further, this concept was rarely communicated to the unit medical sections carrying out the MEDCAP.

Another facet of this same aspect of the problem was that the desired cooperation and the placing of the Vietnamese health care provider in the forefront of a MEDCAP assumes that the Vietnamese personnel were always present. In fact, frequently when line unit medical detachments went out into the hamlets or to visit orphanages, they went alone, with only a Vietnamese interpreter. This was certainly true during tactical operations. The reality was that if no Vietnamese were present as part of the team, it was obviously impossible to funnel the credit to them. As previously noted, MEDCAP was often carried out in more parts of Vietnam where there was no other available medical care.

The ultimate goal of medical assistance programs in Vietnam was to have the Vietnamese themselves capable of maintaining a satisfactory level of preventive and therapeutic medicine. Much was contributed to this aim by the U.S. medical efforts, especially in the MILPHAP and other training programs and in support of the medical school. Conversely, the MEDCAP II program resulted in only temporary relief of the situation and contributed little to the long-term improvement in the health status of the Vietnamese.[59] Americans often preferred to deliver direct care with its more immediate and obvious results and gratification on the part of the care provider, but this was of no benefit developmentally. This failure to achieve permanent benefit was due, in part, to the constantly changing military scene, with units moving into different areas of responsibility and taking their medical sections with them. The programs tended to fluctuate with the tactical situation and availability of medical personnel.[60] Further, the Vietnamese did not have the ability to assume and supply all the programs, especially as the U.S. military presence decreased.

In October 1970, the Committee on Government Operations of the House of Representatives issued a report on the civilian medical program for Vietnam. It concluded the AID's efforts to improve the civilian medical program in Vietnam "have met with only limited success." The construction and establishment of a National Institute of Public Health in Saigon improved public health services. The role of U.S. personnel was limited as they lacked direct authority or responsibility for medical programs; they rendered assistance and served as advisors but had little or no direct authority to take action to correct known deficiencies. AID personnel worked in the GVN MOH in unsatisfactory conditions, caught between the mutually exclusive aims of efficiency and having the GVN personnel appearing to be in control.[61]

Cooperation between USAID and MOH personnel had not succeeded, in part, due to the discrepancy between the salaries of USAID/VN personnel and their GVN counterparts, with the U.S. stipends being substantially greater, resulting in an unequal appearance of authority and importance. Further, the tendency of AID personnel to avoid becoming involved in the detailed operations of the civilian medical program denied their GVN counterparts the opportunity to develop necessary operational capabilities.

Aside from the desire by command to keep the medical units busy, the altruistic inclinations of the medical personnel to help the people around them, and the policy aim of winning the hearts and minds of the people, there was yet another potential reason to carry out these programs. As mentioned earlier, gathering groups of people as occurred on MEDCAPs gave the GVN an opportunity to disseminate information and propaganda. That was a two-way street. It was also an opportunity to gather information and intelligence.

According to the Office of the Surgeon General, a Russian named Leodardov first suggested medical intelligence as a subject field in 1931.[62] The field was recognized by the U.S. Army in 1933, but no action in that regard was taken until 1940 when the task was assigned to the surgeon general. It is notable that during World War I, American forces had had little need for medical intelligence, as operations were limited to areas with a sanitary culture comparable to that of the United States. Further, during the previous two-and-a-half years of war our allies had gained experience that they could share with U.S. forces. A medical intelligence unit was established in April 1941.[63] Early in the 1950s, the agency was taken out of the Preventive Medical Division and established as a separate entity, the Medical Intelligence and Information Agency (MIIA). This agency became part of the Defense Intelligence Agency (DIA) in 1961.[64]

Medical intelligence is an integral part of the intelligence picture and "is absolutely essential in all military operations."[65] Its major function was the collection of data regarding health problems where troops were operating. Without adequate medical intelligence, there is a needlessly high incidence of preventable illness.[66] This form of medical intelligence differs from tactical intelligence that can also be obtained medically. This intelligence was both a byproduct and an aim of all medical activities during the conflict. Both friendly and enemy wounded provided intelligence. S2/G2 reviewed the overall physical condition of prisoners of war (POWs), including the evidence of diseases or malnutrition. Unusual findings as evidence of biological warfare or gas casualties were sought.

MEDCAPs provided a good representation of the general health of the populace.[67] The finding of a strain of malaria endemic to North Vietnam but not South Vietnam indicated an increased presence of North Vietnamese in the area and foretold increased enemy activity. Civic action assistance caused an increase in intelligence data from the villagers.[68] SF Sgt. Maj. Patsy Angelone found that when he was treating wounded VC, they tended to be very talkative. "It was like, as long as I talk, I'll be treated right."[69] Lt. Col. James Lay considered that the "overriding objective" of the program was to obtain intelligence. The quality and quantity of the intelligence was directly proportional to the people's loyalty, support, and confidence in the U.S. unit.[70]

Discussing his unit MEDCAP program, armor officer Capt. John Irving reported intelligence gains by the unit S-2 attributed to the program. "Initially, the S-2 found the people hostile and uncommunicative. The villagers became very cooperative after seeing the positive results of our program." The villagers volunteered the locations of mines placed in the roads. He also commented that the VC were "concerned over our presence and attempted to undo at night what we had accomplished during the day." They made frequent visits to disprove our ability to provide protection.[71] It clearly was a demonstration of the beneficial effect of having a unit remain in one location for a significant period of time.

Charles Webb, a lieutenant colonel in the Medical Corps, also addressed the use of medical services in collection of intelligence. "People under treatment are frequently very cooperative in revealing information about the guerilla force." For this information to be useful, the commander must ensure that the medic is advised by intelligence experts and that the information is promptly processed and not ignored. Further, captured medical supplies can provide useful information about enemy logistical and support capabilities.[72] The collection and study of enemy equipment is a well-recognized intelligence activity, for through such measures much can be learned about enemy resources.[73]

The reporting and use of intelligence garnered during medical civic action appears to have been most common at the small unit level. An example of the benefit of this goodwill was that in one week, children led 25th Division soldiers to seventy-two booby traps and mines.[74] A review of the divisional intelligence summaries for the 25th Division during 1966, 1967, and 1968 contained comments regarding the capture of medical supplies, referenced by the box or by the pound. It noted medical facilities discovered in tunnels and from the air. It cataloged medical documents, some of which verified that the treatment facilities were quite permanent in nature, with patients staying in them up to six months at a time. There were descriptions of medicines and books captured, VC medics killed or captured, and wounded VC being treated and then transferred.

The reports did not indicate, however, that strategic intelligence was obtained during medical civic action programs. In fact, during the entire time reviewed, there was no mention in the intelligence reports of any medical civic action or MEDCAPs by U.S. troops, rather the reports indicated that combat soldiers during their normal activities gathered all the information. A prisoner of war did confirm that sick enemy personnel were being moved into the front lines, which was interpreted as indicating the VC determination to exert maximum effort in the 1968 Spring Offensive.[75]

Either there was no intelligence gathered through medical civic action, it was dealt with on the local, small unit level, or it simply was never recorded. Review of the intelligence reports of the 1st Infantry Division (The Big Red One) for October 1965 through December 1968, and 1st Cavalry Division records from January 1968 to December 1969, contained material similar to that of the 25th Division. There was commentary about captured materials and documents. There was no mention of intelligence from the medical sources or of MEDCAP teams in any of the reports.[76]

Capt. Russel H. Stolfi of the Marine Corps evaluated the marine civic action program in Vietnam. He reported anecdotal instances of intelligence benefits leading to small unit actions as ambushes. While he determined that "the correlation between medical treatments and the erosion of the VC political and military effort was too complex for definition," he also concluded that "the most effective correlation between civic action and the struggle against the VC was information received from the peasants."[77] Intelligence was simply another facet of the civic action and pacification program that is difficult to evaluate in retrospect and was very possibly underutilized.

The United States and the GVN held a different view of the entire pacification program. This difference was illustrated by variations in English and Vietnamese language. The effort had initially been under the *Xay Dung Nong Thon* program, literally "rural construction." The GVN saw this as a giant public works program. In deference to the Americans, in English, it was referred to as the Ministry of Revolutionary Development (MORD), but in Vietnamese the "new" ministry was called *Bo Xay Dung,* or Ministry of Construction. The essential difference between the U.S. and Vietnamese viewpoints was that of a public construction program as opposed to social development.[78]

General Westmoreland and Vietnamese Gen. Nguyen Khanh

discussed civic action within the first six months after Westmoreland assumed his command. The Vietnamese placed less emphasis on civic action than did the U.S. leadership. Khanh stated that "there was nothing new in soldiers assisting civilians but that the matter had not been give much emphasis." In general, it had been confined to helping peasants harvest the crops, "but this had not been possible in recent years because of the war."[79]

One of the means through which the military could work with the nonmilitary was through civic action. This would help discourage popular support for insurgent movements and encourage local populations to assist the military in operations against such movements. Shortly before leaving office, President Eisenhower sent Lt. Col. (later major general) Edward Lansdale to Vietnam on a secret mission to liaison with the CIA. He presented his report in 1961 to President Kennedy and recommended concentration of a strategy of military civic action to regain the support of the population.[80]

President Johnson, in a news conference held at his Texas ranch on 5 July 1966, said he considered the "other war" as crucial to the future of South Vietnam and Southeast Asia as the military struggle. He pointed to the medical school being constructed, which would graduate as many doctors each year as were currently serving the entire civilian population of Vietnam. He said that at that time, "almost 13,000 village health stations have been established and stocked with medicines from the United States."[81]

Brig. Gen. Glenn J. Collins, USARV surgeon, reported in 1968 that the revised MEDCAP II program had increased both the number and scope of projects. "The program has effectively carried modern medicine, dentistry, and veterinary medicine to practically every village and hamlet countrywide, and has contributed greatly to the achievement of U.S. objectives in Vietnam."[82] Improving the health of the population aided in nation building, increased effectiveness of both the people and the military forces, and contributed to removing health risks to U.S. troops.[83]

Emerging nations face great problems in the health arena. These include associated conditions of hunger, poverty, illiteracy, overpopulation, crowded urban conditions, primitive methods of fecal and refuse disposal, and the lack of safe water supplies, all of which foster disease. In his War College study, Lt. Col. James Pope (MC) concluded that military medicine has a strategic role in emerging nations. The activities of military medicine contribute to social, economic, and political stability. Military medicine, therefore, promotes the foreign policy objectives of the United States.[84] Col. John Sheedy (MC) considered that reduced health conditions were one factor making Indochinese nations vulnerable to subversion. He emphatically stated that with the superiority of the United States in medical capabilities "it is possible that increased efforts in this area might exert a positive anti-subversive influence on the war in S.E. Asia."[85] Neither Pope nor Sheedy address the question of who gets the credit for this care or how such care rendered by U.S. forces in uniform can be transferred to another government.

Robert W. Komer, then special assistant to President Johnson, felt that the extent of the public health and medical assistance programs in Vietnam was not generally recognized. He listed the 1.3 million inoculations for cholera, smallpox, plague, and other diseases given in 1965 alone, and the fact that 83 percent of the population was being protected against malaria. Twenty-six surgical suites were constructed in provincial hospitals in 1965, and in the first five months of the year, there were some thirty-five free world medical teams treating patients and performing operations.[86]

Robert Komer subsequently headed CORDS at its inception, with the rank of ambassador. He felt the medical care program should be a "high priority," because it promoted winning the hearts and minds of the Vietnamese. When asked thirty years later if there were long term benefits to the programs, he replied, "Yes, the population was healthier, and more people were capable of working. Beyond that, it is impossible to say."[87] Komer also claimed credit for the Joint Utilization Program (JU) where civilians were treated in Vietnamese military hospitals. He felt the Vietnamese military was pushed into accepting this concept after the U.S. military formalized admitting Vietnamese civilians into U.S. military hospitals.

Efforts to eliminate duplication in the administration of civilian health programs between AID and MACV resulted in the establishment of joint USMACV/AID working committees in 1968. The committees formulated joint plans for hospital construction, medical supply, medical education and training, preventive medicine, and public health. By including military and civilian Vietnamese medical officials as members of the committees, a base was laid for the future assumption of responsibility for these programs by the Vietnamese themselves.[88]

The results of medical civic action are difficult to evaluate. The figures of funds expended and numbers of patients treated are impressive but do not reflect on the quality of medical care provided, the number of "cures" obtained, or the amount of villagers won over to the cause of the GVN. It can be said that they were welcomed into villages and hamlets and appeared to have a beneficial effect in "winning the hearts and minds of the people."[89]

Medical Corps Col. ElRay Jenkins found that the "overall consensus was that the program was a success. Only after the war did opinions change."[90] The hearts and minds of the Vietnamese people were being won. "Success breeds success"; as the U.S. forces increased in number, every battalion or larger unit was encouraged to participate in the program. (In fact, it became a requirement, rather than simply being encouraged.) "Statistics ruled the day."[91] Medical civic actions expanded until 1969 when planning for withdrawal of American personnel and turnover of the function to the Vietnamese ensued. MEDCAP activities then declined steadily and were discontinued in 1972 when funding ceased.

The war was over, and the medical assistance effort had made little impact on the outcome of the conflict. Many individuals received medical care they might not have gotten without the programs, and many Vietnamese medical personnel were trained. Determining if the program was effective in its primary goal, winning the hearts and minds of the populace, has proven to be very difficult. On the surface it would appear that the program did not work well in Vietnam. "Actually, it worked quite well. The problem was that Vietnam was not a low intensity conflict after 1964."[92] It never was from the standpoint of the enemy.

Col. Raymond Bishop felt the psychological results obtained by the MEDCAP II program were even more difficult to assess than the quality and effect of the medical care rendered. Figures of funds expended and numbers treated certainly do not aid in interpretation of the feelings of the population. He concluded that "the mere presence of the MEDCAP II teams must have lent some credence to the premise that the GVN and the U.S. were interested in the welfare of the Vietnamese people."[93] This begs the question of whether demonstrated interest by the United States as indicated by U.S. soldiers in uniform providing the services under the MEDCAP II program in any way transferred to positive feeling by the people in regard to the GVN.

Traditionally, when the U.S. government has been involved in medical humanitarian assistance, it has been through civilian departments and agencies, primarily the Department of State, USAID, and, to a much less degree, the Peace Corps. Some believed that the DOD should "leave well enough alone." Critics of DOD medical programs argued that the basic mission of the military is antithetical to humanitarian assistance and that the civilian groups, both governmental and private, were capable and structured to do that mission.

Similarly, there were those in the DOD who argued that resources diverted to humanitarian assistance should be redirected to the more traditional military mission.[94] Maj. William Holmberg, discussing Marine Corps civic action, warned that "excessive attention to humanitarian programs will ultimately result in a change in the service image beyond that which is conductive to the procurement of fighting men."[95] As Matthew S. Klimow summarized in his discussion of the future of U.S. armed humanitarian assistance, there is a continuing struggle between two streams of American thought "that have continually vied for ascendancy in the twentieth century, idealism and realism."[96]

Although direct patient care is provided, the real interests served by humanitarian civic action are psychological and political.[97] Support forces, including medical, can be used as a separate element in the projection of power.[98] The programs aimed to reinforce the "Clausewitzian trinity" between the people, the government, and the army. "It is now recognized that medical operations in low intensity conflict scenarios represent the most cost effective and least controversial technique for gaining popular support."[99] Too often, the United States has forgotten which army and government were at issue. Psychological operations should aim the best light possible on the host government, not on the United States[100] The emphasis should be on developing capability, not providing service.[101] There can be no long-term benefit to a patient with no development of a health-care delivery system.

As Col. Raymond Bishop noted, "The MEDCAP programs are of considerable psychological value, but only limited medical value, while MILPHAP is contributing significantly to the health of the Vietnamese people."[102] If the aim of the programs is to upgrade medical care of the host nation, the first steps should be to support and enhance existing capabilities such as hospitals and training programs. This is very different from the question of winning the hearts and minds and using medical care to promote U.S. policy.

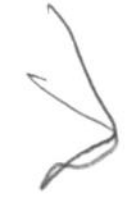

Medical officer David Brown served for five years in Vietnam.

He was on the staff of the assistant director for Public Health of the USAID mission. In his review of his service in Vietnam, he noted a number of difficulties in establishing training programs or a satisfactory health delivery system. The one-year tour prevented adequate institutional memory, with a constant problem of "reinventing the wheel."[103] This was compounded by rotation of Vietnamese counterparts, which meant that established rapport was often of short duration. The Vietnamese government had inadequate money or manpower resources to implement many of the suggestions made by advisors. Programs were instituted before it was determined what the Vietnamese wanted or what they were prepared and able to support. There was never a long-range health plan, making it difficult to set up coordinated long-range assistance programs. Public health and preventive medicine measures directed toward alleviation of the health problems of the bulk of the population who lived in rural areas beyond the reach of the hospital system were largely ineffective. The massive aid program "can thus be regarded as a failure as far as the average Vietnamese has been concerned."[104]

In countries with serious endemic diseases (such as plague or malaria) and the maldistribution of medical manpower and resources permanent changes require long-term commitment. Malnourishment, malaria, and poor sanitation are not cured by an occasional MEDCAP visit. Regardless of the humanitarian intent of alleviating human suffering and misery, in reality, the MEDCAPs accomplished little except to possibly improve the American image. Field commanders did not have the resources to develop health care systems, solve sanitation dilemmas, dig wells, and change lifestyles that had evolved over the centuries. Such activities required a comprehensive strategy and assistance plan beginning with overhauling the health care delivery system of the host nation.[105]

In a 1970 Rand Corporation study, Brian Jenkins noted that "the lack of a clear, attainable, or decisive objective and adequate measures of success in reaching that objective make it difficult to assess the progress of the war in Vietnam. Frequently, increases in the amount of our own military efforts are measured and this is called progress."[106] This was written regarding the entire conflict, but it applies equally to the medical civic action programs as to the combat arms branches. Delivering more doses of medicine does not equate with providing improved medical care.

If the fundamental battle in Vietnam was for the hearts and minds of the peasantry, U.S. hopes for success faced formidable obstacles. In the process of driving the French out of Vietnam, the Vietminh captured the nationalist banner. They drove the white man out, and they appealed to the highest aspirations of the best young Vietnamese of an entire generation. There was no other choice; it was French or Vietminh.[107] Political scientist Hans Morgenthau noted that the government of South Vietnam was "overwhelmingly" composed of men who had sided with the French against their own people, supported in the main by the landowners and the urban middle class. (This was in a country that was overridingly rural in the early 1960s.) The Saigon leadership in the post-Diem period had very thin nationalistic credentials.[108] Historian Ben Kiernan pointed out that winning the hearts and minds among a land-hungry peasant population while propping up the tiny landowning class was wishful thinking.[109] South Vietnamese Gen. Pham Zuan Chieu admitted: "We are very weak politically and without the strong political support of the population which the NLF have."[110] Though the Saigon government did begin a major land reform in 1970, it may well have been too late to gain the support of much of the rural population.

The VC infiltrated the government on a massive scale. The GVN could only govern "with the bayonets of a foreign power" and simply could not compete with Ho Chi Minh and the VC for the allegiance of the people of South Vietnam. No amount of American advice, money, and weapons could overcome that.[111] Journalist Bernard Fall reached the core of the matter at an earlier time, applicable to the period of U.S. involvement, saying, "A thoroughgoing psychological warfare program coupled with effective improvements (good local government, public health, and agricultural reform programs) must provide the local population with a reason to commit itself effectively to the Western side without feeling that it betrays its own national interests."[112]

In a letter to the editor of the *Journal of the American Medical Association,* Dr. Haakon Ragde voiced the opinion that unrealistic planning hindered U.S. medical accomplishments in Vietnam. Much of the effort "attempted to combine the incompatible with the unattainable." Problems were viewed through Western eyes and solutions attempted shaped by Western experience, when improvements rather than solutions were more feasible.[113]

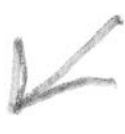

The perverse reality is that the program with the most significant public relations value (MEDCAP) was the least effective in providing long-lasting medical benefit. Certainly some medical good was achieved, and some individuals who received the benefit of reconstruction surgery or correction of congenital deformities such as cleft lip and palate had life-long benefits. For the vast majority of the population, however, medical benefits were minimal and fleeting. While the local populace appreciated these benefits, they did not identify these medical efforts with the government of the Republic of Vietnam. Therefore, these efforts did little to further U.S. foreign policy objectives.[114]

The programs that had the greatest potential for long-term significant health system improvements had little or no publicity or public relations effects. Building a medical school to increase the supply and quality of doctors available to the people of Vietnam had the potential for great long-term benefits. It was a first step in the development of a national system of health care. The MILPHAP program delivered quality medical care, and many Vietnamese civilians derived great and life-long dividends from it. There were significant strides made in upgrading the quality of the Vietnamese physicians, especially among the surgical specialties. The program never received the publicity of the MEDCAPs, either in the United States or in Vietnam.

No tight control of the MEDCAP programs ever existed. Direction from the command level was vague and intermittent. Efforts of the various services such as the marines or the SF were poorly coordinated with the numerically greater army forces, if coordinated at all. Small unit commanders, such as in a battalion, operated under pressure to produce numbers, not to evaluate the programs. A battalion commander needed to improve on the numbers of his predecessor to maximize his OER rating, whether those numbers dealt with numbers of patients treated or enemies killed in action. There was no synergy or significant communication between the small unit MEDCAP programs and the hospital-based MILPHAP or CWCP programs beyond an occasional patient referral with virtually no return feedback to the unit. The potential benefits of the tool of medicine were thus only poorly and partially realized. Some medical benefits were realized, some minor intelligence information was gathered, and some Vietnamese people felt better about the Americans, but the impact was minimal.

There was an almost romantic quality about both the MEDCAPs and the hometown reporting about them. General Westmoreland felt that no program had a more immediate and dramatic effect than the medical civic action program.[115] It was Americans abroad doing good for less fortunate others. It was a person-to-person program where the enlisted soldier could do something to help the needy in a war-torn country. It was GIs giving time, candy, and aid on their own. It was a big military program that could be publicized as something from the grassroots. There were highly trained officers (physicians) involved, but even they seemed to be acting in the best tradition of American medical altruism.

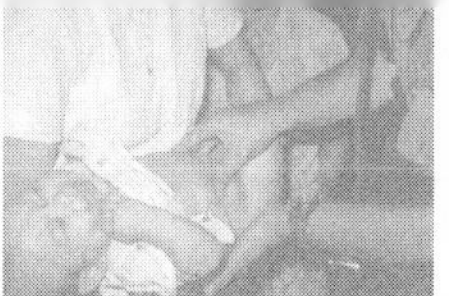

Seven
Conclusions

It is readily apparent that medical civic action in Vietnam had a political motivation. Both the civilian and military leaders used it to advance their aims. While command might have publicized the altruistic elements of the programs, medical benefit to the rural population was truly a secondary consideration. The testimony of medical personnel and my own personal experience suggest this is not how those delivering the care viewed the programs. The doctors, nurses, and corpsmen sincerely felt they were helping the people. They participated in the programs without ulterior motives or even the realization that they were part of a greater plan.

It is of interest to note the difference between how the medical caregivers and those in command evaluated the programs. Without fail, criticism from the physicians, nurses, and corpsmen focused on the quality of medical care delivered, which was substandard. Multiple comments in the reports reflect on the absence of laboratory backup, X-ray availability, and patient follow-up opportunities. In all the monthly reports, end-of-tour reports, and commentaries by physicians and nurses or oral history debriefings, no comments from health care givers refer to the use of medical services as a policy tool. Conversely, reports and memoirs by those at the command level all disregard the quality of medical care delivered and do not even consider it, reflecting favorably on the use of medical care as an instrument of policy.

What can be learned from the American experience in Vietnam about the relationship between medical care and policy? There are many lessons that should be easily discernable. First, to be of lasting value, the programs must train the indigenous population. Otherwise, the programs neither reflect favorably on the host government nor will they remain effective after withdrawal of outside forces. Programs conducted or dominated by U.S. medical units that provide direct care to indigenous civilians provide little long-term value for the host country.[1] After a tour of Vietnam, Israeli Gen. Moshe Dayan remarked that "foreign troops never win the hearts of the people"[2] because care rendered by foreigners in uniform might benefit individuals, but it does not gain support for the host government. Instead, such programs might demonstrate either an inability of the host government to provide for its own people or a lack of enough concern for its own citizens to do so. Medical care for neutral or hostile civilians can also breed resentment among government troops, who see health care being given to less loyal individuals while their own families lack adequate medical care.[3]

Military historian Lewis Sorley maintains that in the final years of U.S. involvement under Gen. Creighton Abrams, there was strong support for the U.S. position and the GVN among the rural population.[4] While many of the programs may have been welcomed by the Vietnamese people, I doubt that the full battle for the hearts and minds of the people was ever won by the GVN.

It is now clear that the United States and the GVN had an uphill fight for the support of the people. The Viet Minh under Ho Chi Minh at the end of World War II had been able to assume the mantle of nationalism. They de-emphasized communist connections. They did not promote those who had supported the French or the Japanese, as did Diem. They were not Catholic. They carefully touted nationalistic aims rather than emphasizing class antagonisms, a strategy advocated by the Moscow-based Comintern and its successor, the Department of Internal Information (*Otdel Myezhdunarodnoi Informatzii* [OMI]).[5] While advocating and positioning themselves as nationalists, they gradually eliminated noncommunist nationalist leaders and solidified control of the country.

The reporting systems for medical care rendered depended on who was being treated. A physician treating U.S. military personnel reported that activity through the army, i.e., USARV (the logistical side of the command structure). If the same surgeon went into the village to care for civilians, he would report that activity to the MACV (the tactical side). Maj. Gen. Spurgeon Neel reported care of U.S. military personnel to the J-4 (Command Supply Organization), whereas he reported MEDCAP and other civilian care activities to the J-3 (Command Operations Division). Neel himself interpreted this as a tactical employment of medical capability to influence the indigenous population.[6] Similarly, physicians assigned to naval and marine units reported care of U.S. military personnel through their command channels to Naval Force, Vietnam (NAVFORV), U.S. Air Force, and USAF Command respectively, while care of civilians was reported to MACV.

There were multiple motivations for the participation in civilian medical care projects. Given the basic inclination of Americans and physicians toward altruism and the provision of humanitarian care, physicians, nurses, dentists, veterinarians, and medics contributed their own time and occasionally funds to caring for needy civilians that demonstrated their compassion for their Vietnamese patients. So, too, did the outpouring of contributions from within the United States. Solicitations aimed at hometown church and civic groups rarely went unheeded.

The second lesson is that civilian care programs were definitely a secondary mission, and throughout the conflict, monthly medical activities reports during periods of significant enemy military activity show either a total cessation or major reduction in medical civic actions.[7] Heavy fighting required the doctors and medical units to attend to their primary mission, caring for the troops. Many programs ceased during and after the 1968 Tet Offensives, never to resume. During the monsoon season when roads became impassable and hindered all travel, medical civic action programs significantly decreased in activity. These fluctuations in the programs made it difficult to convince the people that the programs were going to persist and that their lot was really improving.

On the other hand, the command structure clearly desired to maintain the morale of the medical units and to do so needed to keep the doctors and nurses occupied. By their own writings, Westmoreland and Neel both revealed that they considered doctors with free time to be troublesome. If they were not busy with casualties, then the various civic action programs such as MEDCAP kept them involved providing medical care, which was the only thing they did willingly and well. As one medical services activities report put it, "The MEDCAP II program is a valuable aid in keeping Army medical service (AMEDS) personnel involved in care of patients. Their feeling of being needed is enhanced, at a time when low casualty rates might otherwise lead to idleness and discontent."[8] If there was additional benefit to the recipients and for the strategic situation, it was a bonus. According to Westmoreland and Neel, simply keeping the medical personnel busy would have made the programs a success in and of itself.

Third, medical intelligence is useful. Knowledge of local diseases is essential for this purpose. It aids by keeping friendly troops healthy, off sick call, and available for duty. Medical intelligence also provides information regarding the health and nutrition of the opposing forces, knowledge about the state of its medical facilities, care, and the sophistication and origin of its medicines. In most instances in Vietnam, this collected medical intelligence was discounted or ignored. Warnings about the presence of the enemy emanating from the medical corps based on types of disease not usually seen in the South were rarely heeded.

The available archival records provide no evidence that the medical sections gathered significant tactical intelligence. Knowledge about the state of health of the enemy fighting force was desirable, even though it did not have an impact on operational planning. Information pertaining to evacuation of enemy sick and wounded was used to aid in evaluating the effects of assaults on the enemy logistics system of supply but did not alter U.S. operational planning.[9] Anecdotal reports of possible enemy attacks,[10] booby traps, and ambushes were plentiful, and while this information was used at small unit level, there is no evidence it affected decision making at the command level. Lives were saved by these warnings, but the direction of the war was not significantly altered.

The fourth lesson is that a basic rule of any aid program was not followed in Vietnam. The initiation of programs occurred before determining what the Vietnamese wanted or what they were prepared to support.[11] As Vietnamese General Thang stated, "You are strangers here, and do not understand the people or their problems. You build schools where market places are needed and vice versa, with no regard for the needs or desires of the people."[12] He further indicated that "force fed" civic action programs would not aid the people in developing a sense of pride in the nation. As Maj. Robert Burke pointed out in his discussion of military civic action, a project suggested by the local people is better than one that is "obviously superior" to an outsider.[13]

Gen. Moshe Dayan's criticism was even more severe. He argued doing too much for the Vietnamese administration resulted in both discouragement and loss of confidence by the government and lack of involvement by the population at large.[14] There is little or no benefit to the host country to have U.S. military forces in uniform delivering direct medical care in the countryside. As noted earlier, Brig. Gen. James L. Collins, assistant to the MACV commander, was aware of this problem. "We must not get into position where we overwhelm or compete with the Government of Vietnam."[15] As Col. Allen Keener (SF) concluded, there must be genuine host nation governmental support for civic action of all kinds, and this never existed to a sufficient degree in South Vietnam.[16] Further, as also seen in the combat aspects of the war, the more the foreign troops did, the less inclined the GVN and ARVN were to take on tasks on their own.

The provision of medical care to the needy civilians was beneficial. Unquestionably certain disease categories were more susceptible to these programs than others: skin disorders and acute infectious diseases could be eradicated, war wounds could be healed, broken bones could be set. Immunizations protected many children. Lasting benefit from the correction of congenital deformities, such as cleft lip and palate, clubfoot, congenital hand anomalies, etc., was possible and routinely achieved. Many individuals derived lifelong benefit from the medical aid programs.

The more pressing question is whether the health care system of Vietnam also improved. Ultimately, a program must build an infrastructure to enable the indigenous medical personnel to provide the care. Establishing and developing a medical school in Saigon (now Ho Chi Minh City) and training programs for medical technicians could have increased the number of physicians in the country and improved the health services provided in Vietnamese hospitals. War does not tend to advance social programs. It is ironic but understandable that the long-term programs of education, establishment of schools and training programs, and construction of hospitals and dispensaries garner far less publicity than the direct provision of medical care in the countryside. Many in the countryside may well not know that a new medical school has been created or teachers brought into the country to staff it. They might never know where the additional doctors, nurses, and health care providers came from when they arrive in the villages and hamlets. Further, as the report of Children's Medical Relief International pointed out, for a new institution to survive, it must be "rooted in a national need and willingness" and maintained by a sophisticated local staff trained for its growth.[17]

There was a significant absence of satisfactory long-term planning regarding health care between the GVN and the U.S. civilian and military agencies. The Medical Appraisal Team was unable to discover any long-range plan for USAID-GVN participation in the development of health services, even though it was apparent that the United States was committed to a role in Vietnam for many years. Short-range goals were defined on a yearly basis, in part, for budgetary purposes.[18]

The curtailment of U.S. and FWMAF participation in the war limited the long-term benefits. The lesson here is that short-term medical care is valuable, but the change in a nation's health care system requires time and sustained effort. This is also true when attempting to show a population that the government sincerely wishes to improve the lot of the people, even if aid by outsiders is needed to accomplish the task.

Elementary sanitation measures taught by the SF and navy corpsmen with marine units at the hamlet level had the potential to improve the quality of life in rural areas, without requiring sophisticated equipment or massive infusions of funds. These efforts required constant reiteration and the provision of basic items such as soap and toothbrushes to be effective. In the turmoil of the post-war era with shortages of bare necessities, as well as the political upheaval, it is unlikely that these advances were maintained.

The fifth lesson is that medical care programs can be effective in advancing U.S. strategic aims, under proper circumstances. The programs have proven to be of value in limited rather than full scale wars. Col. ElRay Jenkins (MC) considered medical operations in low intensity conflicts the most cost-effective and least controversial technique for gaining popular support.[19] They are of use in wars of insurrection, as opposed to wars to expel an invader. Programs must be constituted so that they gain support for the host country, rather than for U.S. or other foreign forces. They are of greatest benefit early on, rather than at the end of conflicts or when the level of warfare has been increased.

In a full scale conventional war between major military units, the battle is not for support of the people, but rather to defeat an opposing force. For this reason, winning over the population can only be attempted in a limited war, such as wars of insurrection. In these instances, the true battle is for the support of the people. This situation differs greatly from that which occurred in both world wars, when the occupied countries simply wanted the invaders evicted. There was no need to win over the population. While providing medical care to the people was helpful to them, it did not play a policy role.

In guerilla warfare, support of the population is critical to the success of the insurgency. An outside force can be effective in an insurgency only if the indigenous combatants are at least even.[20] In Vietnam, medical care might have been significant, but only in periods of insurgency. After Tet in 1968 when the character of the war changed with the huge losses sustained by the VC in the South and the fighting passing into the hands of the NVA and certainly at the time of the end game when there was increased invasion of major North Vietnamese units, military medical care for civilians could not have changed the outcome. An accurate recognition of the situation, limited as opposed to total war, must be made before attempting to use medical care as an instrument of policy.

To achieve maximum success, programs should be local and limited, at first, in scope. The local personnel should be featured, rather than the outsiders. U.S. personnel must be "as invisible to the people as possible."[21] Procedures, treatments, medicines, and devices should not be introduced if they cannot be ultimately transferred to local control and maintained after the withdrawal of the outside agents. Teaching should always be carried out, and the local population should be required to participate rather than simply receive care.[22]

According to Surgeon General Leonard D. Heaton, the provision of medical services to the civilians of Vietnam or any other country in which the U.S. military was involved was extremely important. He viewed health services as "a weapon of great power."[23] Medicine was interwoven in our foreign policy.[24] Medical assistance was easily understood by the people, "offering a strong bridge to better understanding" and an appreciation of our sincere intentions.[25] The military has the manpower necessary and is better organized to contribute to nation building through the use of medical services than any other institution.[26] It also possesses the additional significant benefit of being able to provide security for these efforts when necessary.[27]

Constructing schools and training programs can improve an entire health care system if qualified personnel are available to run the programs after withdrawal of the foreign forces. The phrase, *after withdrawal of the foreign forces,* recurs throughout this review. The foreign forces will always leave, eventually. Programs should be planned so that this fact does not negate their impact and make them worthless. It is imperative to train individuals who can later teach to establish a lasting effective program. Teaching the teachers forms the foundation for a durable program. This cannot be accomplished in months or a few years but requires a long-term commitment. It is questionable whether this type of commitment can be made while fighting a war. Programs must be established at a level of sophistication that the host country can maintain and support. Highly technical equipment is useless without skilled technicians, proper maintenance, and basic infrastructure such as adequate electricity. This problem occurred as U.S. Army hospitals were turned over to the ARVN at the time of the U.S. troops' withdrawal. Without the U.S. forces and civilian contractors, there was not adequate power or maintenance capability to run the installations.

Medical Corps Lt. Col. James K. Pope points out that military medicine promotes stability within developing nations by both supporting the army troops in their primary mission and participating in the military assistance program. These latter activities are separate from participation in military civic action.[28] He concludes that military medicine can contribute to social, economic, and political stability and thereby assist in carrying out U.S. foreign policy objectives. This is clearly the political use of medical services.

Military medical units providing medical care to civilians is proper. The medical unit is occupied doing what it does best, caring for the sick and injured. It helps to maintain the proficiency of the unit, and thereby enables it to better perform its primary mission, care of the troops. While there is some difference of opinion about the advisability of fighting units performing civic action,[29] these concerns are not pertinent for a medical unit. Unlike a combat platoon, a medical unit does not need to "turn off" its altruistic tendencies to carry out its primary mission. Instead, physicians, nurses, and corpsmen simply redirect their efforts to the civilian population. The "warrior" mentality vital to the fighting branches need not be maintained within the Medical Corps.[30] Therefore, the considerations as to whether civic action is appropriate activity for a fighting force simply do not apply to a medical unit. In a reversal of the command level position, the political gain in treating civilians is a secondary benefit from the standpoint of the medical personnel, who viewed the medical benefits as primary.

While the gratitude of those receiving medical aid is often readily apparent, it is difficult to measure the unhappiness of those who are denied care. Failure to care for all the sick and injured might breed resentment among the population, which hinders building support for the host nation. If the team moves elsewhere, either by schedule as in ship-based ventures or due to the strategic and combat situation, those left untreated might constitute a core of resentment and disillusionment left behind to fester. Similar strife arises if the team exhausts all its medical supplies before treating everyone who seeks care.[31] This emphasizes the need for long-term rather than itinerant programs and training of the indigenous health providers.

In the United States, itinerant surgery is discouraged. Going into a community to perform operations and then leaving the patient in the care of another, who might not be qualified to handle the complications or postoperative problems involved, is considered a breach of ethics. This might be tolerable in a war situation in regard to hospital surgery and emergency care, but it is less so in regard to the sudden cessation in a clinic or medical program. The patients might view the premature departure of the physicians who were providing care as abandonment, contributing to a degree of disillusionment. The guerrilla or insurgent force can use this lack of permanency to demonstrate the weakness of the government and the fact that they, the guerrillas, are a permanent force while the foreign army is not. In Vietnam, there was an apparent difference in the concern and care of the people's own army and the army of the outside forces. This served to diminish the Vietnamese armed forces in the eyes of the population and certainly did not gain support for the GVN.

A local practitioner of medicine might view a team of foreign physicians descending upon his or her community, performing sophisticated surgical procedures, and then departing, with displeasure. It might leave the impression that the local physician is of marginal quality and training. This loss of "face" or "merit" or standing in the community is especially important in many Asian societies. Furthermore, leaving the physician to manage patients postoperatively is unfair to both the physician and the patient. In an ideal situation, medical programs would have trained the local physician to perform the procedures in question. That is far more expensive, time-consuming, difficult, and less dramatic in its impact. It will, however, create long lasting results.

The preceding chapters have outlined how medical care was

delivered to civilians. It is also apparent that for this care to be effective, either medically or as an instrument of policy, certain criteria must be met, certain conditions must prevail, and the orientation of the programs must be carefully adjusted to maximize results. It is not possible to win the support of the people unless their allegiance is both available and sought after by both sides of the conflict. An invader will not win over the population by using medical care if the populace simply wishes them to be expelled. It is only when both sides seek support of the indigenous population that medical care can help win them for one side or the other.

Even in a limited war, providing medical care will not win the hearts and minds over to the host government and help defeat the insurgency, unless there is a deficiency in the health services available to the people. Provision of an item or service already in abundance would not have a significant effect. For example, in France in World War II there was an intact well established medical care system, even if it faced shortages due to the war. Vietnam had a well documented shortage of physicians, nurses, and other health workers even during peaceful times, let alone during a prolonged war throughout the country.[32] The people needed health services, even if Western medicine may not have been exactly what they desired.

The imbalance between good deeds and the guerillas' willingness to use intimidation, violence, and terror in dealing with civilians magnifies the difficulty in succeeding in pacification. As Brig. Gen. Samuel S. Sumner noted in the Philippine Insurgency Campaign, "Nothing that we can offer in the way of peace or prosperity weighs against the fear of assassination which is prosecuted with relentless vigor against anyone giving aid or information to the government."[33] No civic action campaign can succeed until long-term security can be guaranteed to the population at risk. This security must be present both day and night, a situation that did not exist in most of the Vietnamese countryside during the war.

Another major consideration and a sixth lesson to be learned concerns who gets the credit for the programs. Certainly the United States wishes its servicemen and -women abroad to be welcomed by the citizens of whatever country they are engaged in. There is nothing wrong with gaining favor for U.S. troops among the rural population. But that was not and cannot be a major aim of policy. If the conflict in question is a war of insurrection, then the aim must be to gain support for the government of the host country. As early as 1962–63, it was recognized by the U.S. military that the local populations recognized the medical care came from the Americans and not their own government.[34] In Vietnam, foreigners and outsiders had ruled the country for many years, and the average citizen viewed the government as the enemy.[35]

Military medical care of civilians during wartime might be useful as an instrument of policy, provided that the instrument is wielded correctly. Relative to the costs of warfare, both in manpower and money, it is an extremely cost-effective use of medical personnel. There is benefit to both the givers and recipients on a humanitarian level. It satisfies the command desire to keep the doctors busy. It can, rarely, provide some useful intelligence material, though this aspect of the program is most likely overvalued. It can only be a useful tool in properly selected conflicts, when the underlying situation and status of the medical care system make the provision of medical services a highly desired and needed commodity.

The seventh and final lesson to be learned from the Vietnam experience might be that the failure of command to clearly define and comprehend the nature of the conflict limits the usefulness of medical care as a policy instrument. Civilian policy makers and military commanders must realize the limitations of military medical care for civilians as an instrument of policy. An accurate understanding of the type of conflict being waged is fundamental to making proper decisions regarding the use of military medical aid to civilians.

There is no excuse for expenditures of manpower hours and funds, as well as putting personnel in harm's way, if doing so will not be of benefit to the aims of the United States. This might mean that civilian medical care programs should not be used in a war to expel an invader but limited to use in wars of insurrection and where the real battle is for the support of the people. If used, those participating in the programs must be made to understand their significance and importance from a policy standpoint. The programs must be constructed to be lasting and not interrupted by the movements of troops and units. They must be in support of, rather than in place of, the local caregivers. In spite of this, however, in Vietnam and other conflicts medical care to civilian populations in need of it nourishes the moral being of those giving the care even as it heals the bodies of those receiving it.

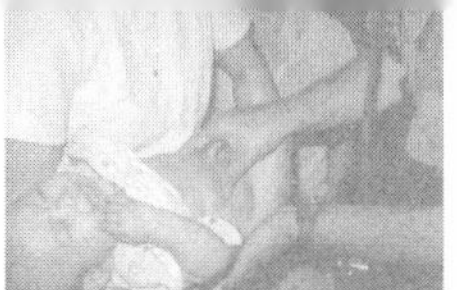

Appendix A
Patients Treated in MEDCAP

Year	*Treatments*
1963	690,119
1964	2,720,898
1965	4,478,158[1]
1966	9,800,783
1967	10,314,113
1968	5,812,544
1969	3,159,616
1970	2,219,715
1971	449,781[2]

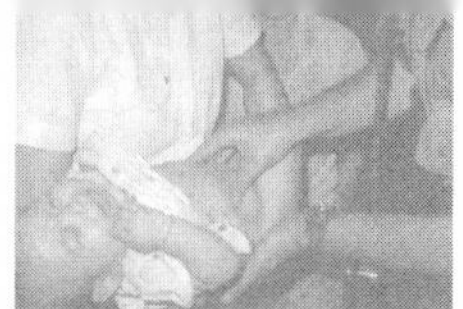

Appendix B
CORDS

United States Military Assistance Command, Vietnam, Directive No. 10-12: Organization and Functions for Civil Operations and Revolutionary Development Support (Saigon: 28 May 1967). The Assistant Chief of Staff for Civil Operations and Revolutionary Development Support (CORDS) is assigned functions as follows:

1. Advises COMUSMACV, MACV staff elements and all U.S. civilian agencies on all aspects of U.S. civil/military support for the Government of Vietnam's Revolutionary Development (RD) Program.
2. In conjunction with Government of Vietnam authorities, develops joint and combined plans, policies, concepts, and programs concerning U.S. civil/military support for RD.
3. Supervises the execution of plans and programs for U.S. civil/military support of Revolutionary Development.
4. Provides advice and assistance to the Government of Vietnam, including the Ministry of Revolutionary Development, the Republic of Vietnam Armed Forces Joint General Staff and other GVN agencies on U.S. civil/military support for Revolutionary Development including U.S. advisory and logistical support.

5. Develops requirements for military and civil assets (U.S. and GVN) to support Revolutionary Development.
6. Serves as the contact point with sponsoring agencies for RD programs. Maintains liaison with sponsoring agencies in representing their interests in civil non-RD programs and activities in the field. Maintains direct operational communications with field elements for these programs.
7. Is responsible for program coordination with the various Mission (USOM) civil agencies in planning and implementation of non-RD activities as they impinge upon or affect RD-related activities.
8. Provides MACV focal point for economic warfare to include population and resources control and for civic action by U.S. forces.
9. Evaluates all civil/military RD activities including provision of security for RD by US/FWMAF/GVN military forces and reports on progress, status, and problems of RD support.
10. Acts on all RD support matters pertaining to subordinate echelons.
11. Directs advisory relationships with GVN on RD and RD-related matters.

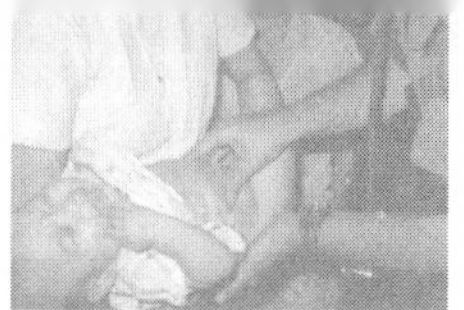

Appendix C
Expenditures

The precise financing of civilian medical care is virtually impossible to ascertain. The multiple organizations involved (USOM, AID, CIA, the military, the embassy, volunteer organizations, such as Project HOPE, CARE, Catholic Relief, churches, etc.) make an accurate accounting extremely difficult. In some instances (like the CIA) the budgets were secret and still are secret. CARE and Catholic Relief supplied hundreds of tons of food, medicine, and materials that do not appear in any military or government budget. Much of the funding was within larger appropriations for all the civic action/pacification programs. Some of the care was delivered using supplies obtained through routine requisitions, rather than those specifically intended for civilian aid programs. Small units like SF teams obtained medical supplies via barter or scrounging. Many units solicited donations from their own members to use in orphanages, hospitals, refugee camps, and on MEDCAPs, as well as having these soldiers appeal for aid from their hometown churches and civic groups. There is no full account of these donations. The following figures can therefore only be viewed as an approximation. They should provide an understanding of the order of magnitude of the programs.

The AID 1962 budget for 1963 for the Far East was

$17,020,400. The entire strategic hamlet program in Vietnam was $22 million, all of which could be considered as civic action.[1]

Under the 1963 MAAG plans, expendable medical supplies for MEDCAP would be funded by AID. Supplies would be distributed through the existing RVNAF medical depot system. When the first teams arrived in the middle of January 1963 (TDY from Japan), arrangements were made to borrow medical equipment from the RVNAF medical depot system. Loan items were replaced as Continental United States (CONUS) shipments arrived. Initial quantities valued at $250,000 for use in MEDCAP were ordered through USOM. The total value for anticipated delivery through December 1964 was $1.081 million. The monthly requirement for each team was approximately $25,000. For 1963, ARVN medical depots issued supplies worth $221,150, and USOM issued $27,402 in the final seven months of the year.[2] During the last half of the 1963 fiscal year (FY 63), the Military Assistance Program (MAP) cost for MEDCAP (the teams totaling 127 military medical personnel) was $34,290 and the USOM cost was $300,000.[3] U.S. civic action assistance for Vietnam during FY 64 was $5.4 million, of which $5.2 million was MAP funds. AID provided $200,000 for medical civic action support.[4] From February 1963 to March 1965, a total cost of expendable medical supplies issued was $1,111,862, for a cost per treatment of $0.24.[5] Funding for MEDCAP was provided by USOM, and supplies were distributed through existing Vietnamese medical depots. Total cost of supplies expended in 1964 was $583,091. This represented $0.22 per treatment.[6]

The total funds expended for MEDCAP issue grew steadily from January 1963 through September 1966.

1963 = $248,552
1964 = $586,091
1965 = $727,219
1966 = $1,182,945 for nine months
(which prorates to $1,623,617 for an entire year)

Adding the eighteen different unit accounts (as II Field Force, 173rd Airborne Brigade, PHILCAGV, 1st Infantry Division, etc.) a total of $354,421.73 MEDCAP II issues for the period July 1965 to September 1966 results.[7] International voluntary agencies provided significant support to US/FWMAF military civic action programs. During the first six months of 1966, the Catholic Relief Services provided in excess of 14,000 tons of food, clothing, and medical items. CARE furnished over $800,000 worth of material and foodstuffs during the same period. Additionally, the State of Hawaii provided the 25th Infantry Division, in Operation Helping Hand, 442 tons of items for distribution to the Vietnamese population.[8] Because U.S. forces were automatically involved in all aspects of the civic action program, they distributed the bulk of the International Voluntary Agency supplies brought into Vietnam. In the first five months of 1966, U.S. forces distributed 12,860 tons of food, clothing, and medical supplies of the Catholic Relief Services and about $760,000 worth of CARE commodities.[9]

The Provincial Health Assistance Program (PHAP) was a multinational assistance effort with two aims: to give direct medical aid to the Vietnamese and to expand Vietnamese capabilities in clinical health care. In FY 67, the financial support for this program amounted to $36 million, and the GVN proposed budget for FY 67 was $1.5 billion.[10]

In December 1966, AID increased the Public Health Division Budget from $26.8 million in FY 66 to $50 million for FY 67 in an effort to place greater emphasis on the civilian medical program. The USAID Budget October 1967 programmed $11,339,400.[11]

Obligations in the public health area for FY 68 and FY 69 were $27.6 million and $20.4 million, respectively. Obligations for FY 70 have been estimated at $17.9 million.[12]

The Government Accounting Office (GAO) estimated that, in FY 68 to FY 70, the equivalent of $85 to $98 million was obligated or budgeted annually for health activities in Vietnam, including medical personnel, medical supplies, and construction or renovation of health facilities. Indirect U.S. assistance in the form of counterpart piaster support went from $3.3 to $1.2 million per year during the same period.[13] This piaster support was not calculated into medical services expenditures. DOD also provided assistance in the form of medical supplies and equipment in support of GVN civilian health programs. DOD obligated about $5.3 million in FY 68 and $6.7 million in FY 69 and had budgeted $9.8 million in FY 70. An additional $26.5 million was obligated by DOD in FY 68 and FY 69 for supply and construction support of the GVN military health programs. DOD had programmed about $18.2 million for supplies in FY 70 in support of the GVN military health program.[14] It has been estimated that from July 1964 through 1969, about $42.8 million was provided by voluntary agencies, international organizations, and other free world countries to the GVN health programs in the form of health teams, medical supplies and equipment, and construction or renovation of health facilities.[15] In 1967, public health programs received the dollar equivalent of about $20.2 million (about 7.2 percent) of the GVN civil budget, including about $3.3 million (4.9 percent) in available counterpart funds.[16]

Ambassador William E. Colby succeeded Robert Komer as head of CORDS. As of December 1969, forty-six countries were providing assistance to Vietnam. Donations and services for economic and social programs, exclusive of the United States, amounted to $125,444,451. There were also upwards of twenty-three voluntary agencies from other free world countries and international NGOs operating programs that assisted refugees and other war victims directly and indirectly. These groups, as well as civilian war casualties, benefited from free world health and medical assistance, which amounted to more than one-third of the total amount—approximately $42,797,185.[17]

In the summer of 1967, a joint working group between USAID and MACV was formed to eliminate duplication of efforts. One example of this was the Joint Construction Committee. On 5 March 1968, MOH and RVNAF approved the concept of joint medical effort. This committee proposed joint planning, construction, staffing, and occupancy of all medical facilities. The original MOH program would have cost $18.5 million; by joint planning, estimated savings were $6 million.[18]

For FY 67 the DA budget for medical support was $600,000. The MEDCAP budget included $5 million from AID, $5 million from MACV, and $5.3 million from the DA. Medical non-MEDCAP aid for the same organizations was $11.5, $13.4, and $14.1 million. The figures remained the same for MEDCAP in 1968, but non-MEDCAP aid decreased to $12.3, $13.8, and $12.8 million.[19] These figures are consistent with the USAID/DOD Project Summary Sheet (15 February 1967) estimated MEDCAP funding for supplies.[20]

A 29 April 1967, joint MACV/USAIDV message directed that each unit submit one requisition for resupply requirements regardless of use, e.g., military or MEDCAP. This was to preclude duplicate supply accounting and material handling at both the depot and unit levels. This required additional funding for all medical depots: an additional $1.8 million to USARPAC to reimburse Army Service Forces (ASF) for issues to United States Army, Vietnam (USARV); an additional $700,000 to Bureau Medicine Project twenty funds for Fleet Marine Force Pacific; and an additional $0.3 million to the 7th Air Force for use by 12th USAF hospital, Cam Ranh Bay.[21] The Military Assistance Command (MACMD) Fact Sheet (21 May 1968) dealing with the Civilian War Casualty Program (CWCP) noted that the initial upgrading of three hospitals would cost $1.7 million with a second stage priced at $3 million.[22] In FY 69, a total of VN $11,540,000 was allocated by the GVN to construct maternity dispensaries and medical centers at refugee sites.[23]

Essentially, the medical AID/DOD realignment program resulted in the U.S. Department of Defense financing 50 percent of the cost of medical supplies and equipment requisitioned by USAID. The program was designed to support various medical programs throughout RVN that were sponsored by the MOH. The following funds were available to USAID from DOD: FY 70 $5,509,000; FY 71 $5,091,000; and FY 72 $5,758,000.[24] In the realignment programs in FY 71, there were ten active projects with a total budget of $80.175 million. For FY 72 the number of active projects was reduced to seven with an approved budget of $58.071 million. In July 1972, the FY 73 program containing five programs with a budget of $36.144 million was approved. For FY 71 (USAID) the MEDCAP initial budget was $2 million, with a final budget of $607,000 of which $503,000 was expanded. For MILPHAP, the figures were $5.3, $6.6, and $5.092 million. For FY 72 (DA), MEDCAP was $600,000 and the MACV-recommended budget was $200,000. The MILPHAP figures were (DA) $5.7 million and (MACV RECCOM) $5.7 million. For FY 73, MILPHAP (DA) was $5.15 million and (MACV RECCOM) $5.15 million.[25]

As is apparent from these figures, the budgetary process was convoluted, confusing, and overlapping among many organizations. Simply totaling the known budgeted expenditures gives a total of $183,887,257 for the duration, not including the FWMAF funds, which easily bring the total to over $350,000,000, or one-third of a billion dollars spent on civilian health care in Vietnam. The expenditures actually most likely exceeded that figure by a significant margin, and an estimate of a total cost of close to half a billion dollars is not unreasonable.

By the middle of 1967, the war was costing $20 billion per year.[26] This figure would rise with the Tet Offensives of 1968, the increased bombing under Nixon, and the reequipping of the ARVN. Department of Defense spending on procurement alone from 1964 to 1969 (inclusive) amounted to $107.6 billion.[27] The total expended on civilian medical care clearly amounted to less than 1 percent of the costs of the war.

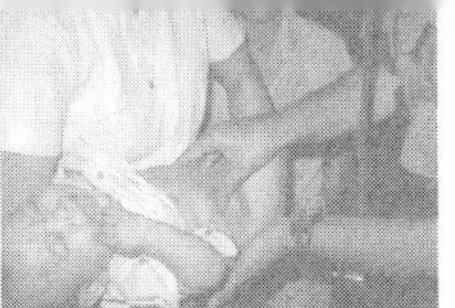

Notes

Chapter One: Introduction

1. James T. Fisher, *Dr. America: The Lives of Thomas A. Dooley 1927–1961* (Amherst: University of Massachusetts Press, 1997).

2. Report from Command Surgeon to Military History Branch, *Medical Civic Action Program (MEDCAP),* MACV Command Overview, 19 March 1972.

3. *Conduct of the War,* Final Report of the Research Project, 68, Center of Military History (hereafter CMH) Box HRC Geog V. Vietnam 319.1, File 228-01.

4. The phrase "hearts and minds" frequently occurs in writings about the war and is a shorthand for all the programs intended to gain support of the peasantry for the GVN, including all of civic action, pacification, rural and then revolutionary development, etc.

5. ElRay Jenkins, "Medical Civic Action Programs (MEDCAP) and Medical Readiness Training Exercises (MEDRETES) as Instruments of Foreign Policy," Military History Institute Archives, Carlisle Barracks, Pa. (hereafter MHIA) U.S. Army War College Student Paper (hereafter Student Paper) AD-A 195 304 (24 May 1988).

6. William C. Westmoreland, *A Soldier Reports* (Garden City, N.Y.: Doubleday, 1976), 267.

7. Telegram from Department of State to embassy in Saigon (25 July 1964) following White House meeting that day with President Johnson, McGeorge Bundy, Robert McNamara, William Bundy, Michael V. Forrestal, Earle G. Wheeler, John T. McNaughton, William E. Colby, and W. Averell Harriman. *Foreign Relations, 1964–68,* vol. 1 (1964; rep., Washington, D.C.: Department

of State, Government Printing Office, 1968), 571–72, National Archives (hereafter NA). "Highest level" is a frequent code for reference to the president of the United States.

8. The development and practice of civil affairs and military government may be traced to George Washington's command in the Revolutionary War. Thomas B. Turner, "Problems of Civilian Health Under War Conditions—General Concepts and Origins," chap. 1 in *Preventive Medicine in World War II, Civil Affairs/Military Government Public Health Activities* (Washington, D.C.: Office of the Surgeon General, 1976), 3.

9. Ibid., 580.

10. Ibid., 4.

11. Edwin A. Rudd, "U.S. Military Role in Civic Actions in Vietnam," MHIA, Student Paper (19 January 1966), 2. Military civic action is defined as "the use of preponderantly indigenous military forces on projects useful to the local population at all levels in such fields as education, training, public works, agriculture, transportation, communications, health, sanitation, and others contributing to economic and social development, which also serve to improve the standing of military forces with the population."

12. The *Hukbong Bayan Laban sa Hapon* (People's Anti-Japanese Army) shortened to Hukbalahap or Huks were Filipino Communist insurgents during and after World War II.

13. Edward G. Lansdale, *In the Midst of Wars: An American's Mission to Southeast Asia* (New York: Harper & Row, 1972), 50–51.

14. Thomas W. Scoville, *Reorganizing for Pacification Support* (Washington, D.C.: Center of Military History, 1991), 3. The definition of pacification is imprecise, "some saw it as controlling the population; others as winning the people's allegiance. Some viewed it as a short-term military operation aimed at quashing opposition; others as a long-term process of bringing, in addition to security, economic, political, and social development to the people."

15. Henry A. Kissinger, "The Viet Nam Negotiations," *Foreign Affairs* 47 (January 1969): 212.

16. Msg. Westmoreland MAH794 to Sharp 311050Z Aug 67, Section 6, 3–4, LBJ Library, NSF, Komer-Leonhart File, Container 15, Folder: MEMOS-The President 1967.

17. Kissinger, "The Viet Nam Negotiations," 213.

18. Ibid., 214–15.

19. Daniel E. Evans Jr. and Charles W. Sasser, *Doc: Platoon Medic* (New York: Pocket Books, 1998), xvii.

20. "21 Military Physicians Killed in Southeast Asia," *U.S. Medicine* (1 January 1972), Naval BUMED Vietnam Files, Folder: Casualties.

21. John L. Cook, *Rescue Under Fire: The Story of Dust Off in Vietnam* (Atglen, Pa.: Schiffer Publishing, 1998), 67.

22. Richard V. N. Ginn, *The History of the U.S. Army Medical Service Corps* (Washington, D.C.: Office of the Surgeon General and Center of Military History, 1997), 321.

23. News Release, Office of the Surgeon General (28 February 1966), NA, Record Group (hereafter RG) 112 Box 64, 3rd Field Hospital.

24. Admiral U.S.G. Sharp, "Report on the War in Vietnam (As of 30 June 1968), 268, Naval BUMED Files, Folder: Code 18; Leonard D. Heaton Papers, MHIA, Senior Officer's Debriefing Program, 2:4:27; Extract Chief Nurses Conference, 44th Medical Brigade (December 1967), NA, RG 472, Box 1, Medical Education and Training Committee, 1968.

25. Nellie L. Henley (18 December 1969), MHIA, Oral History Files, Box 1, File 206-02.1.

26. DA Msg 17 (2 July 1984), Military History Institute Vietnam Room, Carlisle Barracks, Pa. (hereafter MHI-VNR), Folder: Medical #8 Nurses.

27. Marguarite J. Rossi, MHIA, Senior Officer Oral History Program, transcript 24.

28. "We were stopped frequently by the VC and they were wanting some medical supplies. QU: You had to buy your way out? Yes. QU: At that time they didn't want to put your people under? [kill them] No, they wanted the equipment we had, they were getting half of it anyway." MSG Billy J. Akers, SF, MHIA, AMEDDS Oral History Files, Box 1, File 228-01.

29. "Revolutionary Development: Plan for a New Vietnam," MACV Office of Information, Command Information Pamphlet 4-67 (February 1967), 12, NA, RG 112, Box 1, Envelope: Untitled.

30. James H. Forcee, "Medicine—A Concept for Meeting Its World Challenge," *Journal of the American Medical Association* 178 (1961): 153–54.

31. Leonard D. Heaton, *Surgeon General Staff Conference Notes* (7 August 1964), 2, NA, RG 112, Box 9, Folder: Surgeon General Staff Conference Notes, vol. 33 (Bound Copy) 3 Jan 64 – 27 Oct 64.

32. *Conduct of the War,* Final Report of the Research Project, 68, CMH, Box HRC Geog V. Vietnam 319.1, Folder 228-01.

33. Cyrus R. Vance, "Some Current Aspects of the Army Medical Service Mission," Address delivered at annual meeting of the Society of Medical Consultants to the Armed Forces, Walter Reed Army Medical Center (17 November 1963), reprinted in *Military Medicine* 129 (May 1964): 393–96.

34. Bedford H. Berry, "Medicine and United States Foreign Policy: A Partnership for the Seventies," *Military Medicine* 137 (January 1972): 15.

35. Leonard D. Heaton, *Surgeon General Staff Conference Notes* (15 June 1968), NA, RG 112, Box 9, Folder: Surgeon General Staff Conference Notes.

36. Heaton was concerned over both the loss of morale if military people were out of uniform, as well as the protection the uniform offered. Ibid., (31 July 1964), NA, RG 112, Box 9, vol. 33 (Bound Copy), 2.

37. See Warren F. Kimball, *The Juggler: Franklin Roosevelt as Wartime Statesman* (Princeton, N.J.: Princeton University Press, 1991), chap. 7.

38. Col. John L. Beebe, "Civic Action in Vietnam," speech to U.S. Army Civil Affairs School, Ft. Gordon, Ga. (25 May 1963), 1, U.S. Army Troop Information Support Unit No. 6-3-63, CMH, Geog V. Vietnam Drawer 388.5, Folder: Civil Affairs.

39. U. Alexis Johnson, "The U.S. and Southeast Asia," *Department of State Bulletin* 48 (29 April 1963): 640.

40. Frances FitzGerald, *Fire in the Lake* (New York: Random House, 1972), 330.

41. Summary History of MACV, Military History Branch, HQ MACV (12 March 1970), 2, CMH, Drawer: Geog V. Vietnam 319.1, Folder: 229.01 HRC Geog V. Vietnam 322 MACV.

42. William P. Bundy, "The Path to Vietnam," *Department of State Bulletin* 166 (4 September 1967): 7.

43. Ibid., 187. For a full discussion of the Battle of Ap Bac, see Neil Sheehan, *A Bright Shining Lie: John Paul Vann and America in Vietnam* (New York: Random House, 1988).

44. Commentary by Stanley Karnow, "Some Lessons and Non-Lessons of Vietnam, A Conference Report," Woodrow Wilson Center (7–8 January 1983), 24.

45. Bundy, "Path to Vietnam," 8.

46. Karnow, "Some Lessons and Non-Lessons of Vietnam," 24.

Chapter Two: Previous Use of Medical Care for Foreign Civilians

1. Fitzhugh Mullan, *Plagues and Politics: The Story of the United States Public Health Service* (New York: Basic Books, 1989); Leonard A. Scheele, "Military Medicine and the U. S. Public Health Service," *The Military Surgeon* 114 (January 1954): 37–40.

2. Scheele, "Military Medicine and the U.S. Public Health Service," 37.

3. Maj. Azel Ames, in discussing Franklin Kemp's "Field Work in the Philippines," noted the paper's theory that the only way to prevent diseases within the army was to take care of the people around the troops. *Proc. Annual Meeting Association of Military Surgeons of the U.S.* 9 (1900): 73–85.

4. George R. Bentley, *A History of the Freedmen's Bureau* (Philadelphia: University of Pennsylvania, 1955); Herman Belz, "The Freedmen's Bureau Act of 1865 and the Principle of No Discrimination According to Color," *Civil War History* 21 (1975): 197–217; Robert H. Bremmer, "The Impact of the Civil War on Philanthropy and Social Welfare," *Civil War History* 12 (1966): 293–303; Todd L. Savitt, "Politics in Medicine: The Georgia Freedmen's Bureau and the Organization of Health Care, 1865–1866," *Civil War History* 28 (1983): 45–64; Martin Abbott, *The Freedmen's Bureau in South Carolina, 1865–1873* (Chapel Hill: University of North Carolina Press, 1967); Barry A. Crouch, *The Freedmen's Bureau and Black Texans* (Austin: University of Texas Press, 1992); Randy Finley, *From Slavery to Uncertain Freedom: The Freedmen's Bureau in Arkansas, 1865–1869* (Fayetteville: University of Arkansas Press, 1996); William L. Richter, *Overreached on All Sides: The Freedmen's Bureau Administrators in Texas, 1965–1868* (College Station: Texas A&M Press, 1991); and Howard White, *The Freedmen's Bureau in Louisiana* (Baton Rouge: Louisiana State University Press, 1970).

5. Charles H. Mitchell IV, "The Medic as an Instrument of National Policy or What in the World is the Department of Defense Doing in Medical Humanitarian Assistance?" MHIA, Student Paper AD-A 234 134 (8 April 1991), 6.

6. Graham A. Cosmos, *An Army for Empire: The United States Army in the Spanish American War* (Shippensburg, Pa.: White Mane Publishing, 1994); John M. Gibson, *The Life of General William C. Gorgas* (Durham: Duke University Press, 1950); Mary C. Gillette, *The Army Medical Department 1865–1917* (Washington, D.C.: Center of Military History, 1995); William J. Lyster, "The Army Surgeon in the Philippines," *Journal American Medical Association* 36 (5 January 1901): 30–34; John Morgan Gates, *Schoolbooks and Krags: The United States Army in the Philippines, 1898–1902* (Westport, Conn.: Greenwood Press, 1973), 59.

7. Gates, *Schoolbooks and Krags,* 270.

8. Gillette, *Army Medical Department 1865–1917.*

9. Gates, *Schoolbooks and Krags.*

10. Kemp, "Field Work in the Philippines," 73–85; William J. Lyster, "The Army Surgeon in the Philippines," 30–34.

11. Sanitation was absent with human and animal waste disposal in close proximity to the houses. Force was used to change these conditions, ensuring penning of the animals, relocation of waste disposal sites, and creation of clean water sources. See G. E. Meyer, "The Massacre of Balangiga," 3, NA,

RG 319, Folder 37, History File 1 Jan–31 June [*sic*] 1917; George D. DeShon, Memoir, 1890–1913, DTD February 15, 1913, The George D. DeShon Papers, MHIA.

12. Mitchell, "Medic as an Instrument of National Policy," 8.

13. Andrew J. Birtle, *U.S. Army Counterinsurgency and Contingency Operations Doctrine 1860–1941* (Washington, D.C.: Center of Military History, 1998), 48.

14. Gillette, *Army Medical Department, 1865–1917,* 216.

15. Leonard R. Friedman, "American Medicine as a Military-Political Weapon," *Military Medicine* 131 (October 1966): 1275.

16. Crawford W. Sams, *"Medic": The Mission of an American Army Doctor in Occupied Japan and Wartime Korea* (Armonk, N.Y.: M.E. Sharpe, 1998), 206.

17. John F. Taylor and Jerry L. Fields, "Health Care as an Instrument of Foreign Policy," MHIA, Student Paper AD-A 149 434 (9 May 1984), 12–13; James W. Hendley, "Health Services as an Instrument of United States Foreign Policy Toward Lesser Developed Nations" (Ph.D. diss., University of Iowa, 1971), 372–73; Floyd L. Wergeland, "Army Medical Service in Korea," *Military Review* 36 (September 1956): 60.

18. Sams, *"Medic,"* 212, 215.

19. Albert E. Cowdrey, *The Medic's War: United States Army in the Korean War* (Washington, D.C.: Center of Military History, U.S. Army, 1987).

20. NA, RG 319 Records of the Army Staff Box 41, Folder: Annotated Bibliography-Lessons Learned VN [Folder 520, 2 of 3].

21. James B. Shuler, "Medical Practice with the Marines on Occupation Duty in Korea," *U.S. Armed Forces Medical Journal* 7 (1956): 1040–50; Wergeland, "Army Medical Service in Korea," 58–64; Wallis L. Craddock, "United States Medical Programs in South Vietnam: Hope for the Free World," MHIA, Student paper 705 29 (3 October 1969), 2.

22. This study focuses on medical care that is a component of civic action. For a general discussion of pacification, see Richard A. Hunt, *Pacification: The American Struggle for Vietnam's Hearts and Minds* (Boulder, Colo.: Westview Press, 1995).

23. For a discussion of the Ho Chi Minh Trail, see John Prados, *The Bloody Road: The Ho Chi Minh Trail and the Vietnam War* (New York: John Wiley & Sons, 1998).

24. Leo Heiman, "Guerrilla Warfare: An Analysis," *Military Review* 43 (July 1963): 34.

25. David G. Marr, *Vietnam 1945: The Quest for Power* (Berkeley and Los Angeles: University of California Press, 1995), 81.

26. For Africa see Merideth Turshen, "The Impact of Colonialism on Health and Health Services in Tanzania," *International Journal of Health Services* 7 (1 November 1977): 7–35. Health services were determined by the economic, social, and political requirements of German and British colonial rulers, rather than by the health needs of the African population; Terence O. Ranger, "Godly Medicine: The Ambiguities of Medical Mission in Southeast Tanzania, 1900–1945," *Social Science Medicine* 15B (1981): 262–77; Ann Beck, "Problems of British Medical Administration in East Africa Between 1900 and 1930," *Bulletin History of Medicine* 36 (1962): 275–83; Ann Beck, "The Role of Medicine in German East Africa," *Bulletin of History of Medicine* 45 (1971) 170–78; Judith N. Lasker, "The Role of Health Services in Colonial Rule: The Case of the Ivory Coast," *Culture, Medicine and Psychiatry* 1 (1977): 277–97. The native's gratitude toward the doctor creates for France unlimited rights to the land of Africa; David Arnold, ed., *Imperial Medicine and Indigenous Societies* (Manchester: Manchester University Press, 1988). The administration of health policies is complex. Medicine was itself a primary vehicle for imperial ideas and their application; Patrick A. Twumasi, "Colonialism and International Health: A Study in Social Change in Ghana," *Social Science Medicine* 15B (1981): 147–51. For the Indian subcontinent, see L. C. A. Knowles, *The Economic Development of the British Overseas Empire* (New York: Albert & Charles Boni, 1925); Poonam Bala, *Imperialism and Medicine in Bengal: A Socio-Historical Perspective* (Newbury Park, Calif.: Sage Publications, 1992); David Arnold, *Colonizing the Body: State Medicine and Epidemic Disease in Nineteenth-Century India* (Berkeley and Los Angles: University of California Press, 1993); Chee Heng Leng, "Health Status and the Development of Health Services in a Colonial State: The Case of British Malaya," *International Journal of Health Services* 12 (1982): 397–417.

27. Lawrence Freedman, *Kennedy's Wars: Berlin, Cuba, Laos, and Vietnam* (New York: Oxford University Press, 2000): 289.

28. Robert H. Slover, "This is Military Civic Action," *Army* 13 (July 1963): 48–49.

29. "The Military believed that the threat still came from classical cross-border aggression involving substantial armies, and that if forces were developed for these contingencies, they could probably cope quite well with guerilla campaigns. They did not believe that the reverse was true." Freedman, *Kennedy's Wars,* 290.

30. Raymond H. Bishop Jr., "Medical Support of Stability Operations: A Vietnam Case Study," MHIA, Student Paper 690 21C (18 February 1969), 5.

31. Danny R. Ragland, "The Role of Veterinary Medical Civic Action in

the Low Intensity Conflict Environment," Command and General Staff College, Fort Leavenworth, Kansas, Student Paper AD-A 198 089 (1988), 30.

Chapter Three: The Ad Hoc or Informal Programs

1. C. Marshall Lee Jr., "Surgical Care of Civilians in Viet Nam," *American Journal of Surgery* 114 (December 1967): 811–12.

2. Alister Brass, "Foreign Medical Aid to South Vietnam," *New England Journal of Medicine* 277 (12 October 1967): 790.

3. Delores E. Fiedler, "Medical Care in Vietnam," *Occupational Health Nursing* 17 (March 1969): 20–22; Charles R. Webb Jr. Medical Newsletter, Office of the Surgeon, Ft. Bragg, N.C. (1 June 1967), 4, NA, RG 319, Box 32, Folder: Surgeon's Newsletter.

4. For an excellent review of this topic of Vietnamese medicine, see Claudius F. Mayer, "Vietnam Medicine," *The Military Surgeon* 115 (September 1954): 198–205. Other worthwhile commentaries include Harvey H. Smith et al., *Area Handbook for South Vietnam* (Washington, D.C.: U.S. Government Printing Office, 1967); David N. Gilbert and Jerome H. Greenberg, "Vietnam: Preventive Medicine Orientation," *Military Medicine* 132 (October 1967): 769–90.

5. Gilbert and Greenberg, "Vietnam: Preventive Medicine Orientation," 774; Frederick M. Burkle Jr., "Delta Med: 'A Fitting Memorial,'" *U.S. Naval Institute Proceedings* (November 1970): 37; Dan C. Cavanaugh et al., "Some Observations of the Current Plague Outbreak in the Republic of Vietnam," *American Journal of Public Health* 58 (April 1968): 742–52; J. D. Marshall Jr., et al., "Plague in Vietnam 1965–1966," *American Journal of Epidemiology* 86 (1967): 603–16; M. B. Miller et al., "Inpatient Medical Civic Action Program at the 12th USAF Hospital, Cam Ranh Bay, South Vietnam," *Military Medicine* 137 (April 1972): 156–58.

6. John A. Sheedy (Col., MC), "Problems Facing Medical Personnel in Counterinsurgency Programs in Southeast Asia," MHIA, Student Paper 661 64X (19 January 1966), 11. Also cited by Richard S. Dobson (Maj., MSC), *USARV Medical Bulletin* (November–December 1968): 46. Neither list the exact location or date of the occurrence.

7. Howard A. Rusk, "The Future Belongs to Those Who Accomplish the Most for Humanity," *Rhode Island Medical Journal* 50 (August 1967): 540.

8. For an excellent discussion of Vietnamese intrafamily relationships and roles, see Neil L. Jamieson, *Understanding Vietnam* (Berkeley: University of California Press, 1993).

9. Bard Van Chantford, "Junior Tom Dooleys: Corpsmen Care for Sick Vietnamese," News Release 3633 (19 December 1969), 3, Naval BUMED Files, Folder: Newspaper Clippings and News Releases.

10. Brig. Gen. Glenn J. Collins, MC, Debriefing (1 August 1968), B-2, NA, RG 112, Box 1.

11. Keith Dahlberg, "Introducing Present-Day Medicine Into Southeast Asia," *Postgraduate Medicine* 40 (December 1966): A-142.

12. "Medical Newsletter," HQ U.S. Army John F. Kennedy Center for Special Warfare (Airborne) Ft. Bragg, N.C. (1 April 1967), NA, RG 319, Box 32, Folder: Surgeon's Newsletter.

13. "Operation About Face," *U.S. Navy Medicine* 57 (May 1971): 47.

14. George A. Carver Jr., "The Real Revolution in South Viet Nam," *Foreign Affairs* 43 (April 1965): 391.

15. Col. F. P. Serong, Report to Gen. Paul D. Harkins, COMUSMACV (October 1962), 42, NA, RG 319, Box 37, Folder: #1 History Backup, 30 Mar 1962–Nov 1963, Folder 498 [2 of 2].

16. Fiedler, "Medical Care in Vietnam," 20; Calvin C. Chapman, "Comprehensive Medical Care in Vietnam," *Archives of Environmental Health* 17 (July 1968): 21; Burkle, "Delta Med," 39; MACCORDS, Implications of Vietnamization on Civilian Health Programs, MHI-Viet Nam Room, Folder: 2034 CORDS.

17. Ralph Levin, End of Tour Report (16 January 1966), Team #10, Tam Ky, NA, RG 112, Box 1; David W. Stickney, "Vietnamese Province Hospital in the War Zone," *Hospitals* 41 (1 October 1967): 70.

18. Fiedler, "Medical Care in Vietnam," 22.

19. Glenn W. Dunnington, MHIA, Oral History Collection, Box 10, File 228-01 (20 May 1969).

20. Serong, Report to Gen. Paul D. Harkins.

21. Hendrick Smith, "More Health Aid for Saigon Urged," *New York Times*, 22 September 1967, 3.

22. David McK. Rioch, "Summary of Certain Observations and Conclusions," (Visit 21 March–9 April 1964), 4, NA, RG 319, Box 38, Folder: #3 History Backup 17 Feb–30 April 1964, Folder 500; Paul B. Lewis, MHIA, AMEDDS Oral History Collection, Box 17, 228-01 (26 March 1976).

23. Jeffrey Greenhut, "I Have Your Wounded," ms, chap. 10, Uniformed Services Medical Library, Rockville, Md., (22 October 1986), 16.

24. Ambassador Maxwell Taylor, Memorandum for the Record (March 31, 1965). *Foreign Relations, 1964–68, Volume II* (Washington, D.C.: Department of State, 1968), 499; Neil Sheehan, "Tribal Revolt Stirs Vietnam Highlands but Fails," *New York Times* (20 December 1965), 2.

25. Arturo Gonzalez Jr., "Unsung Hero of Vietnam: The G.I. Medic," *Today's Health* 41 (1963): 29.

26. Kissinger, "The Viet Nam Negotiations," 212.

27. "Medical Civic Action Program (MEDCAP)," MAAG Vietnam 1963, NA, RG 319, Box 33, Folder: MAAG, USOM Vietnam 1963/2 USAID.

28. Col. Clyde R. Russell, CO 7th SF, "Nuggets from the Special Forces Lode," *Army* 12 (March 1962): 40–41.

29. Det A-502 Monthly Operational Summary (2 June 1967), NA, RG 319, Box 17, Folder: Det A-502.

30. Lt. Col. R. E. Adams, Information Brief: U.S. Army Medical Aspects of Special Forces in the Republic of Vietnam, Office of the Surgeon General (20 November 1964), NA, RG 319, Box 8, Folder: Inform Book COSA visit Far East and Pacific.

31. Gonzalez, "Unsung Hero of Vietnam," 28.

32. L. Richard Morgan, MHIA, AMEDDS Oral History Collection, Box 20, File 228-01, File 228-02.

33. "Doctor Helps VN Boy Walk," *Army Reporter*, 12 August 1967, 1.

34. "Charlie," of course, was the slang term for the Viet Cong or VC: V for Victor, C for Charlie. Charles H. Bartley, MHIA, AMEDDS Oral History Collection, Box 2, File 228-01.

35. David G. Tittsworth, MHIA, AMEDDS Oral History Collection, Box 27, File 228-01.

36. Scott S. Herbert, MHIA, AMEDDS Oral History Collection, Box 13, File 228-01.

37. Barry Zindel, MHIA, AMEDDS Oral History Collection, Box 29, File 228-01; Herbert, MHIA, AMEDDS Oral History Collection, Box 13, File 228-01.

38. Bartley, MHIA, AMEDDS Oral History Collection, Box 2, File 228-01, p. 37.

39. James Whitener, MHIA, AMEDDS Oral History Collection, Box 29, File 228-01.

40. Minutes of the Surgeon General's early morning conference (26 Nov 65), NA, RG 112, Box 10, Oct 65 to Nov 1967, Bound Volume 36 (1 October 1965–18 February 1966).

41. Joe L. Stackard, "Plague, Cholera and Enteric Diseases in Civilian Communities," *USARV Medical Newsletter* 1 (March 1966): 2.

42. James Alford, MHIA, AMEDDS Oral History Collection, Box 1, File 228-01.

43. Valentine B. Sky, MHIA, AMEDDS Oral History Collection, Box 24, File 228-01.

44. Herbert, MHIA, AMEDDS Oral History Collection, Box 13, File 228-01.

45. Whitner, MHIA, AMEDDS Oral History Collection, Box 29, File 228-01.

46. Ibid.

47. Gonzalez, "Unsung Hero of Vietnam," 29.

48. Henry F. Shelly III, MHIA, AMEDDS Oral History Collection, Box 24, File 228-01.

49. Gerald W. Foy, MHIA, AMEDDS Oral History Collection, Box 11, File 228-01.

50. Ibid.

51. Peter Brush, "Interservice Rivalry in I Corps," *Vietnam* 12 (October 1999): 25.

52. Jack Shulimson, Leonard A. Blasiol, Charles R. Smith, and David A. Dawson, *U.S. Marines in Vietnam: The Defining Year 1968* (Washington, D.C.: History and Museums Division, Headquarters, U.S. Marine Corps, 1997), 2.

53. Brush, "Interservice Rivalry in I Corps," 25.

54. William C. Westmoreland, Historical Notes, 8 December 1965: "The Marines have become so infatuated with securing real estate and in civic action that their forces have become dispersed and they have been hesitant to conduct offensive operations except along the coast line where amphibious maneuvers could be used with Naval gunfire support which is available. Over the last several months, this matter has been discussed with General Walt and I have written two letters to him emphasizing the importance of having adequate reserves to take the fight to the enemy." MHIA, Westmoreland Papers, Box 27, Folder: History File 2, Oct 25 to Dec 20, 1965.

55. Shulimson et al., *U.S. Marines in Vietnam,* 13; John M. Mecklin, "An Alternative Strategy for Vietnam," *Fortune* (April 1968): 98; Westmoreland Papers, 8 December 1965, MHIA, Box 27, Folder: History File 2, Oct 25 to Dec 20, 1965.

56. Memorandum, General Staff Council Meeting of 5 July 1966 (8 July 1966), Office of the Chief of Staff, Army, NA, RG 319, Box 14, Folder: General Staff Council Meetings 1960–1967 (1).

57. Michael A. Hennessy, *Strategy in Vietnam: The Marines and Revolutionary Warfare in I Corps, 1965–1972* (Westport, Conn.: Praeger, 1997), 75; Shulimson et al., *U.S. Marines in Vietnam,* 13.

58. Jim Seaton, "A Political-Warrior Model: The Combined Action Program," *Armed Forces and Society* 20 (Summer 1994): 549–63; Edward G. Lansdale, "Civic Action Helps Counter the Guerilla Threat," *Army Information Digest* 17 (June 1962): 51.

59. Mecklin, "An Alternative Strategy for Vietnam," 98; also see Brush, "Interservice Rivalry in I Corps," 22–28.

60. Douglas S. Blaufarb, *The Counterinsurgency Era* (New York: Free Press, 1977), 257–58; Andrew F. Krepinevich, *The Army and Vietnam* (Baltimore, Md: Johns Hopkins University Press, 1986) 174–75.

61. Shulimson et al., *U.S. Marines in Vietnam,* 13.

62. The marines are under the secretary of the navy. John H. Chafee, statement before Defense Subcommittee of the Committee on Appropriations, U.S. Senate (March 17, 1971), MHIA, *Selected Statements on Vietnam by DoD and Other Administrative Officials,* prepared by the Air Force for Department of Defense, 151.

63. "One of the most ingenious innovations developed in the Vietnam." William Westmoreland, *A Soldier Reports* (Garden City, N.Y.: Doubleday, 1976), 165–66.

64. Chapman, "Comprehensive Medical Care in Vietnam," 22.

65. "Hospital Ship in Saigon," *New York Times* (15 September 1966), 40.

66. "Philippine Civic Action in South Vietnam," MACJO 3 (25 December 1971), MHI-VNR, Folder: 2031.4, Philippine Civic Action in S. Vietnam.

67. Combed Committee Evaluation of the Philippine Civic Action Group, Vietnam (PHILCAGV), 10–20 November 1967, NA, RG 319, Records of the Army Staff, Box 23, Folder: COMUSMACV Signature File Jan 1968.

68. "The Medical Program in Vietnam," USAID (5 September 1967), NA, RG 319, Box 38, Folder: USAID Medical Programs.

69. Westmoreland, *Report on the War,* 251.

70. Johnson to Westmoreland, WDC Message 4802, NA, RG 319, Box 13, Folder: Message Files COMUSMACV 1 Apr–30 June 1967, Folder 364.

71. Wheeler to Sharp (CINCPAC) and Westmoreland, JCS Message 6339-66, 17 October 1966, NA, RG 319, Box 13, Folder: Message Files COMUSMACV 1 Oct–31 Dec 1966, Folder 362 [2 of 2].

72. FONECON between General Wheeler and General Westmoreland, 31 December 1969, NA, RG 319, Box 24, Folder: Close Hold Communications, April–December 1969, Folder 444.

73. National Security Action Memo 362, Responsibility for U.S. Role in Pacification (Revolutionary Development), (9 May 1967).

74. James K. McCollum, "The CORDS Pacification Organization in Vietnam: A Civilian-Military Effort," *Armed Forces and Society* 10 (Fall 1983): 111.

75. Westmoreland insisted on the designation *deputy to* rather than *deputy of* to ensure that under no circumstances could the civilian head of CORDS be in command of MACV troops in the absence of COMUSMACV.

76. Scoville, *Reorganizing for Pacification Support,* 54.

77. Robert W. Komer, "Impact of Pacification on Insurgency in South Vietnam," delivered at 66th Annual Meeting of The American Political Science Association, Los Angeles, 8–12 September 1970, Rand Corporation, P-4443, 11.

78. Brig. Gen. Philip Bolté, "Winning Hearts and Minds," *Vietnam* (February 1994): 23–29.

79. Hans Halberstadt, *War Stories of the Green Berets* (Osceola, Wis.: Motorbooks International, 1994), 143.

80. Robert W. Komer, "Clear, Hold and Rebuild," *Army* 20 (May 1970): 19.

81. James K. McCollum, "CORDS, Matrix for Peace in Vietnam," *Army* 32 (July 1982): 48–53.

82. John M. Mecklin, "An Alternative Strategy for Vietnam," *Fortune* (April 1968): 99.

83. Hunt, *Pacification*, 269.

Chapter Four: Formal MEDCAP, CAP, MILPHAP, and CWCP

1. Paul S. Boyer, *Promises to Keep: The United States since World War II*, 2d ed. (Boston: Houghton Mifflin, 1999), 181.

2. Jenkins, "Medical Civic Action Programs," 3.

3. Taylor and Fields, "Health Care as an Instrument of Foreign Policy," 4.

4. Editorial, "Ship of Hope," *Saturday Review* 47 (28 March 1964): 18. One reason for the prevalence of polio, especially in rural areas, was the lack of adequate electricity and refrigeration that are necessary for the storage of the polio vaccines.

5. "U.S. Doctors Spend Christmas Helping Wounded in Saigon," *New York Times* (25 December 1964), 14.

6. Floyd W. Baker, "Medical Assistance to the Vietnamese," *USARV Medical Bulletin* 2 (November–December 1967): 10. David G. Eisner, "Medical Civic Action Programs (MEDCAP)," *USARV Medical Bulletin* (October–December 1966): 27.

7. Howard A. Rusk, "The Other War in Vietnam," *Readers Digest* 89 (July 1966): 112. Morris Kaplan, "U.S. Woman Doctor is Running a Hospital for Ill Montagnards," *New York Times* (10 July 1966), 4.

8. "Some Factors that Influence the Rural Health Program in Vietnam," MAAG Vietnam, 2 NA, RG 319, Box 33, Folder: MAAG, USOM Vietnam 1963/2, USAID.

9. Col. F. P. Serong arrived in Vietnam on 31 July 1962, with two years experience fighting the Communist insurgency in Burma. He was the former commandant of the Jungle Warfare Training Center in Canunga, Queensland. He was seconded as special advisor in Counterinsurgency to Gen. Paul

Harkins, COMUSMACV. The Australians were under the operational control of MACV.

10. Col. F. P. Serong, report to Gen. Paul D. Harkins, "Current Operations in South Vietnam," October 1962, 42, NA, RG 319, Box 37, Folder: #1 History Backup, 30 March 1962–November 1963, Folder 498 [2 of 2].

11. "Provincial Health Assistance Project (PHAP)," NA, RG 112, Box 92, Folder: Medical Programs.

12. William C. Moncrief Jr., "The Provincial Health Assistance Program in the Republic of Vietnam," *USARV Medical Bulletin* 2 (Jan.–Feb. 1967): 39.

13. Spurgeon Neel, *Medical Support of the U.S. Army in Vietnam 1965–1970* (Washington, D.C.: Department of the Army, 1991), 162.

14. MACV Directive 40-20, 8 December 1968, NA, RG 112, Box 86, Folder: Subject Files 1960–1969 MACV Directives.

15. J. W. Humphreys Jr., "End of Tour Report," USAID/Saigon (1 May 1967), 2–3, NA, RG 319, Box 38, Folder: USAID Medical Programs.

16. Ibid., 5.

17. "Medical Civic Action Program," NA, RG 112, Folder: Medical Civic Action Program (MEDCAP); Memorandum 40-5, HQ MAAGV (14 June 1963). On 21 November 1962, the Office of the U.S. Secretary of Defense approved the recommended U.S. Medical Civic Action Program (MEDCAP) for Republic of Vietnam. The program was implemented 27 January 1963. NA, RG 319, Box 33, Folder: MAAG, USOM Vietnam 1963/2 USAID.

18. "Some Factors that Influence the Rural Health Program in Vietnam," 2.

19. "Medical Civic Action Program," NA, RG 112, Folder: Medical Civic Action Program (MEDCAP).

20. B. F. Black, Memorandum: Intensification of Civic Action Programs in Republic of Vietnam, J55/Memo/008-63 (30 September 1963), NA, RG 319, Box 38, Folder: #2 History Backup January 1964–4 February 1964, Folder 499.

21. "Some Factors that Influence the Rural Health Program in Vietnam," 4.

22. USMACV Office of the Command Surgeon, "Medical Service in the Republic of Vietnam, January 1970–April 1972," III-8, MHIA, AMEDDS Oral History Medical Records Collection, Box 3.

23. "MEDCAP Requisitions," COMUSMACV to SECDEF, MACV 18247 (27 May 1966), NA, RG 112, Box 90, Folder: 228-02 Historians Sources Files, Medical Civic Action Program 1965–1967.

24. Bishop, "Medical Support of Stability Operations," 15.

25. Army Medical Serves Activities Report, USMACV, 1964, NA, RG 112, Box 83, Folder: USARV-Military Assistance Command.

26. Neel, *Medical Support of the U.S. Army in Vietnam,* 164.

27. President Lyndon B. Johnson, "Southeast Asia Aid Program," Read at news conference at the White House June 1, 1965, repr., *Department of State Bulletin* 52 (June 28, 1965): 1054–56.

28. "Text of President's Message on Funds for Vietnam," *New York Times* (5 May 1965), 18.

29. Greenhut, "I Have Your Wounded," 8.

30. H. R. McMaster, *Dereliction of Duty: Lyndon Johnson, Robert McNamara, The Joint Chiefs of Staff, and the Lies that Led to Vietnam* (New York: Harper Collins, 1997).

31. "(a) OBSERVATION: Medical Civic Action Programs are not always properly planned, coordinated, and scheduled. (b) EVALUATION: Frequently one particular village or hamlet may be served by many different agencies while others are totally neglected. MEDCAPs are not always scheduled on a regular basis and often are sporadic in nature. Patients may be treated for the same ailment many times within the span of several days. Generally patient records are not kept by personnel in charge of MEDCAPs." Operational Report-Lessons Learned, 29th Civil Affairs Company, period ending 31 October 1969. "A not infrequent problem was duplication of effort despite all the concurrence and approvals required to initiate a MEDCAP II program. An example of this occurred in a small orphanage in the village of Hiep Hoa, near Bien Hoa. It was discovered that a MEDCAP II team from II Field Force visited the orphanage on Tuesdays, an Air Force team on Thursdays, and a team from the 173rd Airborne Brigade on Saturdays. This was accidentally discovered when one of the teams switched their MEDCAP day and arrived at the orphanage to find another team holding "sick call." Each of the three teams had proper documentation for conducting MEDCAP in the orphanage." Each was totally unaware of the activities of the other teams. The anecdote is undated. Bishop, "Medical Support of Stability Operations," 19.

32. Alfred R. Kitts, "Pacification Can Work," MHIA, Student Paper AD-A 774 234 (31 October 1970), 6.

33. "A Monthly Medical Civic Action Activity Report (RCS CICNPAC 6000-1) will be prepared as of midnight of the last day of the month, using MACV Form 303, dated 26 August 1965." MACV Directive 40-9, (28 December 1965), 2, NA, RG 112, Box 89, Folder: Subject Files 1960–1969 Medical Care—Medical Civilian Assistance Program—Vietnam.

34. USARV Regulation 40-39, 29 August 1967.

35. John F. Reed, MHIA, AMEDDS Oral History Collection, Box 23, File 228-01, 16.

36. Rev. Calvin Thielman to the president (27 July 1966), LBJ Library,

NSF, Komer-Leonhart Collection, Container #14, Folder: Medical Relief [2 of 2].

37. Army Medical Service Activities Report, 52nd Artillery Group, 26 January 1967, NA, RG 319, Box 91, Folder: USARV-52nd Artillery Group 1960–69.

38. 1st Battalion, 8th Artillery Army Medical Services Activities Report 12 February 1969, NA, RG 112, Box 78, Folder: USARV-1st Battalion, 8th Artillery 1960–69.

39. 14th Infantry, 25th Division Army Medical Services Activities Report 7 February 1970, NA, RG 112, Box 78, Folder: USARV-2nd Battalion, 14th Infantry, 25th Division 1960–69.

40. Bishop, "Medical Support of Stability Operations," 18.

41. 44th Medical Brigade Regulation 40-9, 31 July 1968.

42. "On average 30 bars of soap are passed out to villagers per MEDCAP along with pamphlets explaining how to use it." Army Medical Service Report, 2nd Battalion, 12 Infantry (11 February 1969), NA, RG 112, Box 78, Folder: USARV-2nd Battalion, 12th Infantry 1960–69.

43. Directive 40-9, HQ USMACV, 28 December 1965.

44. Mitchell, "Medic as an Instrument of National Policy," 16.

45. James A. Wier, MHIA, AMEDDS Oral History Collection, Box 29, File 228-01, Folder 206-02.1, 62.

46. Al Hemingway, *Our War Was Different: Marine Combined Action Platoons in Vietnam* (Annapolis, Md: Naval Institute Press, 1994), 3.

47. Ibid.

48. Ibid.

49. Seaton, "A Political-Warrior Model," 550.

50. Shulimson et al., *U.S. Marines in Vietnam,* 621; Hennessy, *Strategy in Vietnam,* 168.

51. D. L. Evans Jr., "USMC Civil Affairs in Vietnam," *Marine Corps Gazette* 52 (March 1968): 24.

52. Charles R. Anderson, *Vietnam: The Other War* (Novato, Calif.: Presidio Press, 1982), 68.

53. 4th Marines MEDCAP, 3rd Marine Division, Combat Information Bureau, III Marine Amphibious Force, Da Nang Press Center (26 June 1969), Naval BUMED Files, Folder: Newspaper clippings and news releases.

54. Lewis W. Walt, *Strange War, Strange Strategy* (New York: Funk & Wagnalls, 1970), 32.

55. Fortunately, classes at the medical school were taught in English. Release No. 280-66, Combat Information Center, III Marine Amphibious Force, Da Nang Press Center (23 February 1966), Naval BUMED Files, Folder: Newspaper clippings and news releases.

56. William D. Parker, *U.S. Marine Corps Civil Affairs in I Corps Republic of South Vietnam April 1966–April 1967* (Washington, D.C.: Historical Division, Headquarters, U.S. Marine Corps, 1970), 42.

57. Russel H. Stolfi, *U.S. Marine Corps Civic Action Efforts in Vietnam March 1965–March 1966* (Washington, D.C.: Historical Branch, Headquarters U.S. Marine Corps, 1968), 23–26.

58. Joshua Menkes and Raymond G. Jones, "Pacification in Vietnam: A Survey (U)," (Arlington, Va.: Institute for Defense Analyses, Science and Technology Division, December 1967), 27–28.

59. "Disease Keeps Pace with Vietnam War," *Journal of the American Medical Association* 203 (26 February 1968): 23.

60. Medical Situation Report, III Marine Amphibious Force, MACV (13 July 1966), Naval BUMED Vietnam Files, Folder: 3rd MARDIV Medical Support; Dan C. Cavanaugh et al., "Some Observations on the Current Plague Outbreak in the Republic of Vietnam," 742–52; E. James Feeley and John J. Kriz, "Plague Meningitis in an American Serviceman," *Journal of the American Medical Association* 191 (1 February 1965): 412–13.

61. Baker, "Medical Assistance to the Vietnamese," 10–13.

62. "Medical Civic Action Program (MEDCAP)," 5, NA, RG 112, Records of the Surgeon General (Army) 1960–69, Folder: Subject Files 1960–69, MEDICAL CIVIC ACTION PROGRAM (MEDCAP); "Higher authority has directed this program to be substantial in size and effort; that it will have high priority for all three Service medical services." "U.S. Military Provincial Hospital Assistance Program (MILPHAP) Republic of Vietnam," Medical Survey—Vietnam, Report No. 20, 25 June 1965. NA, RG 319, Box 38, Folder: MILPHAP.

63. Norman S. Paul, memorandum for the secretaries of the army, the navy, and the air force, Subject: Military Mobile Medical Teams (10 September 1965), NA, RG 319, Box 31, Folder: AMEDD Aspects of Stability Operations July 67.

64. Greenhut, "I Have Your Wounded," 19.

65. "Just two days ago we dispatched General C. L. Milburn Jr., Deputy Surgeon General of the Army, to assist U.S. representatives in Vietnam in formulating an expanded program of medical assistance for the people of Vietnam. We are contemplating the expansion of existing programs under which mobile medical teams travel throughout the countryside providing on the spot medical facilities, treatment, and training in rural areas." "Text of President's Message on Funds for Vietnam," *New York Times* (5 May 1965) 18.

66. Office of the Surgeon, MACV, Medical Activities Report 1965, NA, RG 319, Box 33, Folder: Medical Activities Report 1965.

67. "U.S. Military Provincial Hospital Assistance Program (MILPHAP)

Republic of Vietnam," Report No. 20, p. 1, NA, RG 112, Box 95, Folder: Military Hospital Assistance Program (MILPHAP).

68. MACV/USAID Joint Directive 4-65, HQ MACV/USOM, 20 December 1965; MACV/USAID Joint Directive 2-67, HQ MACV/USAID, 21 January 1967.

69. Brig. Gen. J. W. Humphreys Jr. and Col. George F. Rumer, "U.S. Military Provincial Hospital Assistance Program (MILPHAP) Republic of Vietnam," 5, NA, RG 112, Box 95, Folder: Military Hospital Assistance Program (MILPHAP).

70. Bishop, "Medical Support of Stability Operations," 27.

71. Ibid., 27.

72. American Medical Association brochure, *Volunteer Physicians for Viet Nam* (Chicago: n.p., n.d.).

73. USMACV, Office of the Command Surgeon, Medical Service in the Republic of Vietnam January 1970–April 1972, Chapter III-23, MHIA, AMEDDS Oral History Medical Records Collection, Box 3, File 228-01.

74. For a good discussion of these cultural differences and social nuances that Americans were often unaware of or ignored, see Jamieson, *Understanding Vietnam.*

75. Kissinger, "The Viet Nam Negotiations," 220.

76. "Medical Civic Action Program," 6.

77. MACV/USAID Joint Directive 2-67 Military Health Assistance program (MILPHAP), 21 January 1967; MACV/USAID Joint Directive, 4-65, HQ MACV/USOM, 20 December 1965.

78. "CENTO UNCLASSIFIED: COUNTER INSURGENCY," NA, RG 319, Box 33, Folder: MACV, USOM Vietnam 1963/2 USAID.

79. "Reorganization of the MACV Medical Advisory Effort," December 1968, NA, RG 319, Box 32, Folder: Reorganizing MACV Advisory Effort 1969—Medical.

80. "U.S. Military Provincial Hospital Assistance Programs (MILPHAP) Republic of Vietnam," Medical Survey Report No. 20, p 5, NA, RG 319, Box 38, Folder: MILPHAP.

81. D. N. Mangravite, End of Tour Report, Advisory Team 71, MILPHAP Team 8 (12 November 1970), Naval BUMED Files, Folder: MILPHAP.

82. Bishop, "Medical Support of Stability Operations," 33.

83. Terry A. Hammes, MHIA, AMEDDS Oral History Collection, Box 13, File 228-01, Folder: 206-02.1.

84. Report to the Subcommittee to Investigate Problems Connected with Refugees and Escapees Committee on the Judiciary, U.S. Senate, "Civilian Health and War-Related Casualty Program in Vietnam," (9 November 1970), 12, NA, RG 319, Box 33, Folder: Civilian War Casualties (45).

85. Progress Report (30 December 1967), 5, LBJ Library, NSF, Komer-Leonhart File, Container 14, Folder: Medical Relief [1 of 2].

86. W. D. McGlasson, "The War within a War," *The National Guardsman* 22 (December 1968): 11; John W. Batdorf and Kirk V. Cammack, "Civilian Casualties in Vietnam," *Rocky Mountain Medical Journal* 66 (March 1969): 46.

87. Letter *Terre Des Hommes* to President Johnson (14 December 1965); *Vietnam Bulletin* issued by British Vietnam Committee (April 1966); Memorandum from American Embassy Saigon to American Embassy Bern (28 May 1966); Memorandum from Richard Holbroke to Komer (20 July 1966), LBJ Library, NSF, Komer-Leonhart Collection, Container #14, Folder: Medical Relief [2 of 2].

88. "The casualty estimates used by the Kennedy subcommittee were extrapolated from USAID and U.S. Military hospital admissions data. As a rule of thumb, one part of the formula consisted of taking the recorded hospital admission figures and doubling it. Subcommittee investigators justified this increase by saying that for every one recorded admission one casualty went unrecorded because of private medical treatment or no treatment at all. In addition, one-third to one-fourth more of the doubled figure was then added as killed outright or died before reaching a medical treatment facility . . . The rationale for these arbitrary increase was not clearly stated." Final Report of the Research Project, *Conduct of the War in Vietnam* (May 1971), CMH, Drawer: HRC Geog V. Vietnam 314.7 to 319.1, Folder: 319.1 Conduct of the War in Vietnam, 71. No data available was submitted to support these alterations in the figures. John Vann letter to COMUSMACV (n.d.). MHIA, The John Vann Papers, File: Kennedy Visit File.

89. Dahlberg, "Introducing Present-Day Medicine Into Rural Southeast Asia," A-142.

90. Department of State Telegram 04284 from American Embassy Saigon to Secretary of State, Washington D.C. (24 March 1971), NA, RG 319, Box 33, Folder: Civilian War Casualties (45).

91. "Civilian War Casualties," MACMD Fact Sheet, 23 May 1968, NA, RG 319, Box 40, Folder: Fact book—COMUSMACV folder 516.

92. "We have no method, and we doubt that one is available under existing circumstances of war, to state with accuracy the number of persons who suffer war-related injuries and receive no treatment, particularly those injured by the Viet Cong in remote areas." MSG State 42966, Rusk to American Embassy Saigon (240347Z Sep 67). LBJ Library, NSF, Komer-Leonhart File, Container #14, Folder: Medical Relief, [1 of 2].

93. Minutes of Medical Policy and Coordinating Committee, U.S.

Embassy, USAID Mission to Vietnam, 14 February 1967, 3, NA, RG 112, Box 95, Folder: Military Hospital Assistance Program (MILPHAP).

94. "Civilian War Casualties Estimated at 4000 per Month. Probably More than Half are Inflicted by the VC." Memorandum from G. D. Jacobson, mission coordinator, to General Westmoreland et al., Embassy of the U.S.A. (25 July 1967), NA, RG 319, Box 31, Folder: #19 History File 6 July 3–August 1967, Folder 475.

95. Matthew J. Harvey, director, congressional liaison, to Senator Edward M. Kennedy (14 January 1971), NA, RG 319 Records of the Army Staff, Box 33, Folder: Civilian War Casualties [45].

96. "Combat Operations: Minimizing Non-Combatant Battle Casualties," MACV Directive No. 525-3 (7 September 1965), NA, RG 319, Box 26, Folder: #1 History File 19 August 24–October 1965, Folder 458 [1 of 2].

97. Harassment and interdiction fire (H&I) was artillery fire into areas of suspected enemy activity without specific knowledge of enemy presence. It was, therefore, by definition relatively blind and indiscriminate. It was instituted under the command of General Westmoreland, and it was curtailed almost totally by Gen. Creighton Abrams when he succeeded Westmoreland as MACV commander.

98. *Conduct of the War in Vietnam,* Final Report of the Research Project (May 1971), 67, CMH, Drawer: HRC Geog V. Vietnam 314.7 to 319.1, Folder: 319.1 Conduct of the War in Vietnam.

99. Civilian War Casualties in the Republic of Vietnam (RVN), Talking Paper (14 April 1971), NA, RG 319, Box 24, Folder: Close Hold Communications 1971, Folder 446.

100. "Support is to include medical and dental care for US Military forces, US civilians as authorized, International Military Assistance personnel to the extent authorized by current regulations and agreements, and civilians for life saving or humanitarian reasons within capability." HQ USMACV Directive 40-5 (9 August 1965), NA, RG 319, Box 32, Folder: MACV Directive 40-5, 9 August 1965.

101. News Release, Office of Assistant Secretary of Defense (Public Affairs) No. 762-67, 16 August 1967, "Three Vietnamese Hospitals to be Constructed for Vietnamese Civilians," Naval BUMED Vietnam Files Folder: Newspaper Clippings and News Releases.

102. JCS 00330, General Wheeler, CJCS, to General Westmoreland, COMUSMACV, 11 January 1968, NA, RG 319, Box 15, Folder: Message files COMUSMACV, 1–31 January 1968, Folder 376.

103. Again, for a discussion of family life in Vietnam, see Jamieson, *Understanding Vietnam.* Life in Vietnam revolved around the family, and many people had never gone more than twenty or thirty miles from their

homes. Since a family often slept two or more in a bed at home, many patients were unwilling to stay in a hospital without a family member. *Conduct of the War in Vietnam,* 67.

104. Lt. Col. John Bullard (MSC), "U.S. Civil Assistance Programs in SVN" Fact Sheet (29 April 1971), 3, CMH, Drawer: HRG Geog V. Vietnam 334 to 370.2, Folder: 228.01 Geog V. Vietnam 350 Travel Pack.

105. ". . . the recommendation that the military civilian casualty hospitals be scrapped in favor of annexes to existing hospitals, will meet with resistance." Memorandum, Peter R. Rosenblatt to Ambassador William Leonhart, SUBJECT: Medical Appraisal Team Report (6 October 1967). LBJ Library, NSF, Komer-Leonhart File, Container #14, Folder: Medical Relief [1 of 2].

106. In this regard it should also be noted that medical regulating policy was to maintain approximately 40 percent bed availability in U.S. hospitals to have the beds available in case of mass casualties. "DOD Support of Vietnam's Civilian War Casualty Program," (undated talking paper), NA, RG 319, Box 33, Folder: Civilian War Casualties (45).

107. Ibid. The concept of joint utilization had been proposed to the Vietnamese by Ambassador Robert Komer, director of CORDS. The ARVN major general in charge of medical services refused the request. Three weeks after the American hospitals promoted and began joint military/civilian occupancy the Vietnamese reversed themselves. Komer considered this to be one of his more significant accomplishments in Vietnam. (Ambassador Robert Komer, interview by author, telephone interview, 17 February 1996.)

108. The initial bed allotment of 1,100 in 1968 was reduced to 600 for 1969 and 1970 and the first eight months of 1971, further then reduced to 400 and finally 200 for 1971 and 1972. Civilian War Casualty Program, "MACV Command Overview" (8 March 1972), NA, RG 319, Records of the Army Staff, Box 33, Folder: MACV-Surgeon-CMD Overview.

109. "Medical Newsletter," HQ U.S. Army John F. Kennedy Center for Special Warfare (Airborne) Ft. Bragg, N.C. (1 April 1967), NA, RG 319, Box 32, Folder: Surgeon's Newsletter. "It is traditional that one should die at home; and it is a common occurrence that a patient who is very ill in the hospital, and being cared for in part by his family, will be removed during the night from the hospital, without permission, to allow him to die at home." "Report of the Medical Appraisal Team to Vietnam" (20 September 1967), 25, LBJ Library, NSF, Komer-Leonhard File, Container #14, Folder: Medical Relief [1 of 2].

110. Lieutenant Colonel Schopper, "Civilian War Casualties in the Republic of Vietnam (RVN)" Talking Paper (26 April 1971), 4, CMH, Drawer: HRG Geog V. Vietnam 334 to 370.2, Folder: 228.01 Geog V Vietnam 350 Travel Pack.

111. Lt. Col. John Bullard (MSC), "U.S. Civil Assistance Programs in SVN Fact Sheet," (29 April 1971), 3, CMH, Drawer: HRG Geog V. Vietnam 334-370.2, Folder: 228.-1 Geog V. Vietnam 350 Travel Pack.

112. "Treatment of Vietnamese Civilian Nations in US Army Military Medical Facilities," HQ 3rd Field Hospital (12 September 1967) Reference USARV Regulation 40-11 and 44th Medical Brigade Regulation 40-44, NA, RG 112, Box 94, Folder: AVBJ-GD-FA Treatment of Vietnamese Civilians in US Army Medical Facilities; MACV Directive 40-14, HQ USMACV (10 January 1968). Reiterated in MACV Directive 40-2, HQ USMAVC (30 September 1971). Change 1, Directive 40-14, USMACV (1 March 1969). USARV Reg No. 4058, Appendix II: Civilian War Casualty Program (CWCP), 10 December 1969, NA, RG 112, Box 78, Folder: USARV Surgeon 1960–69.

113. Army Medical Department Activities Report CY 72, NA, RG 319, Box 69, Folder: 1st Cavalry Division, USARV. p. 15.

Chapter Five: Medical Evaluation of the Programs

1. Joseph E. Brown, "Medic in Enemy Country: But Navy Corpsman Wins Friends in Viet Village," *San Diego Union* (7 April 1966) A-15.

2. Edward B. Glick, "Military Civic Action: Thorny Art of the Peace Keepers," *Army* 17 (September 1967): 67–70.

3. "Doctor Helps VN Boy Walk."

4. Nat Dell, "MEDCAP: Missions of Mercy," *Army Digest* 23 (December 1968): 57–59.

5. Lawrence P. Metcalf, "The CAP Corpsman," *U.S. Navy Medicine Newsletter* 56 (December 1970): 6–19; "One Million Patients for Amphibious Force Medics," *U.S. Navy Newsletter* 54 (December 1969): 40–42; G.D. Despiegler, "NSA Hospital, DaNang, Vietnam," *U.S. Navy Medical Newsletter* 56 (August 1970): 28–30.

6. David Sherman, "One Man's CAP," *Marine Corps Gazette* 73 (February 1989): 57–62.

7. Robert P. Everett, "Seagoing Medcap," *Airman* 13 (December 1969): 60–62.

8. "MEDCAP Team Thaws Icy Vietnamese Village," *The Screaming Eagle* (16 August 1967): 3.

9. Ibid., 3.

10. Advisory Team 100 (MACV) Semi-Monthly Report (18 December 1964) 2, NA, RG 319, Box 39, Folder: #11 History Backup 7 Dec–31 Dec 1964, Folder 509.

11. Peter B. Cramblet, "U.S. Medical Imperatives for Low Intensity Conflict," MHIA, Student Paper AD-A 236 817 (5 April 1991), 8.

12. All Operational Reports-Lessons Learned are located in the Military History Institute Vietnam Room (MHI-VNR), Carlisle Barracks, Pa., under the heading: U.S. Army 11th Cav.

13. Wallis L. Craddock (Col., MC), "United States Medical Programs in South Vietnam," *Military Medicine* 135 (March 1970): 186–91.

14. USARV Surgeon Daily Staff Journal (31 August 1967), NA, RG 472, Box 2, Folder: USARV Surgeon July–September 1967.

15. 1st Battalion, 502nd Infantry Army Medical Services Report (26 February 1968), NA, RG 112, Box 78, Folder: USARV-1st Battalion, 502nd Infantry.

16. Lam Son was the birthplace of Le Loi, a 15th Century Vietnamese hero, and was a code name prefix for many ARVN ground forces operations, as in Lam Son 719 in 1971, which was an attempt to cut the Ho Chi Minh Trail in Laos. 1st Infantry Division, Operational Report-Lessons Learned 1 May to 31 July 1966, MHI-VNR.

17. 1st Cavalry Division (Airmobile) Army Medical Services Report (3 March 1966), NA, RG 112, Box 88, Folder: USARV-1st Air Cavalry Division 1960–69.

18. 11th Combat Aviation Battalion, Operational Report-Lessons Learned 1 May to 31 July 1966, MHI-VNR.

19. "Medical Civic Action Program," *Quarterly Newsletter,* 3rd Field Hospital (10 October 1967): 4, NA, RG 112, Box 80.

20. 58th Medical Battalion Army Medical Service Activities Report (1 January to 31 December 1968), NA, RG 112, Box 80, Folder: USARV Battalions-58th Medical 1960–69.

21. 4th Battalion, 9th Infantry Army Medical Service Activities Report (1968), NA, RG 112, Box 79, Folder: USARV-4th Battalion, 9th Infantry 1960–69.

22. 1st Battalion, 5th Infantry Army Medical Service Activities Report (14 February 1968), NA, RG 112, Box 78, Folder: USARV-1st Battalion, 5th Infantry 1960–69.

23. 4th Battalion, 23rd Infantry (MECH), 25th Division Army Medical Service Activities Report (1968), NA, RG 112, Box 79, Folder: USARV-3rd Battalion, 24th Infantry 1960–69.

24. 2nd Battalion, 34th Armor, 25th Infantry Division Army Medical Service Activities Report (5 February 1967), NA, RG 112, Box 79, Folder: USARV-2nd Battalion, 34th Armor 1960–69.

25. Ibid.

26. 2nd Battalion, 13th Artillery Army Medical Services Activities Report (5 February 1968), NA, RG 112, Box 78, Folder: USARV-2nd Battalion 13th Artillery.

27. 2nd Battalion, 22nd Infantry Army Medical Services Activities Report

(1 February 1968), NA, RG 112, Box 78, Folder: USARV-2nd Battalion, 22nd Infantry 1960–69.

28. 2nd Howitzer, 17th Artillery Army Medical Services Activities Report (4 February 1967), NA, RG 112, Box 78, Folder USARV-2nd Howitzer, 17th Artillery 1960–69.

29. James E. Anderson Jr., "The Field Experience of a Medical Civic Action Team in South Viet Nam," *Military Medicine* 129 (November 1964): 1052.

30. Joseph R. Territo, "How Effective is Your Participation in the Civilian Health Assistance Programs?" *USARV Medical Bulletin* (September–October 1969): 37.

31. John P. Irving III, "The 'Other War'?" *Armor* (May–June 1968): 24.

32. Bishop, "Medical Support of Stability Operations," 11.

33. "Reaction of the Medical Personnel," MAAG Vietnam 1963, 3, NA, RG 319, Box 33, Folder: MAAG, USOM Vietnam 1963/2 USAID.

34. 2nd Battalion, 12 Infantry Army Medical Service Activities Report (11 February 1969), NA, RG 112, Box 78, Folder: USARV-2nd Battalion, 12th Infantry 1960–69.

35. William F. Gast, 1968 Annual Army Medical Service Report (13 February 1969) 2nd Battalion, 77th Field Artillery, 3, NA, RG 112, Box 79, Folder: USARV 2nd Battalion, 77th Artillery 1960–69.

36. 1st Battalion, 27th Infantry Arm Medical Service Activities Report (27 May 1969), NA, RG 112, Box 78, Folder: 1st Battalion, 27th Infantry 1960–69.

37. Naval Forces Vietnam Monthly Historical Summary (March 1966), 26.

38. Commander, U.S. Naval Forces, Vietnam, to Commander, Amphibious Forces, U.S. Pacific Fleet, Naval Forces Vietnam Monthly Historical Summary (May 1966), 42–45.

39. "Junior Tom Dooleys: Corpsmen Care for Sick Vietnamese," Release No. 3633 (19 December 1969), Naval BUMED Vietnam Files, Folder: Newspaper Clippings and News Releases.

40. 1st Battalion, 12th Cavalry Army Medical Service Activities Report (1966), NA, RG 112, Box 78, Folder: USARV-1st Battalion, 12th Cavalry 1960–69.

41. 2nd Battalion, 3rd Infantry Army Medical Service Activity Report (1967), NA, RG 112, Box 79, Folder: USARV-2nd Battalion, 3rd Infantry 1960–69.

42. Ran L. Phillips, (22 November 1968), MHIA, AMEDDS Oral History Collection, Box 22, File 228-01.

43. 1st Howitzer, 40th Artillery Army Medical Service Activities Report (5 February 1968), NA, RG 112, Box 78, Folder: 1st Howitzer, 4th Artillery 1960–69.

44. 1st Battalion, 44th Artillery Army Medical Services Activity Report (8 February 1968), NA, RG 112, Box 78, Folder: USARV-1st Battalion, 44th Artillery 1960–69.

45. "Some Factors That Influence the Rural Health Program in Vietnam," MAAG Vietnam 1963, 9, NA, RG 319, Box 33, Folder: MAAG, USOM Vietnam 1963/2 USAID.

46. Ibid., 9.

47. Bishop, "Medical Support of Stability Operations," 9.

48. "Confusion Concerning Primary Objective of Medical Civic Action," MAAG Vietnam 1963, 1, NA, RG 319, Box 33, Folder: MAAG USOM Vietnam 1963/2 USAID.

49. Army Medical Service Activities Report, USARV-20th Engineer Brigade, 1969, NA, RG 112, Box 82, Folder: USARV-20th Engineer Brigade 1960–69.

50. MHIA, Oral History Interviews, Box 1, File 228-01.

51. Lowell J. Rubin, "Medcap with the Montagnards, *USARV Medical Bulletin* (May–June 1968): 31.

52. Ralph Levin, Captain, MC, Report of Team #10, Tam Ky (16 June 1966), NA, RG 112.

53. Robert J. Wilensky, Capt., MC, Army Medical Service Activities Report (24 January 1968) 588th Engineer Battalion, 20th Engineer Brigade, NA, RG 112, Box 81, Folder: USARV-588th Engineer Battalion 1960–69.

54. 2nd Battalion, 12th Infantry, Army Medical Service Activities Report (11 February 1969), NA, RG 112, Box 78, Folder: USARV-2nd Battalion, 12th Infantry 1960–69.

55. Americal Division, Army Medical Service Activities Report, (28 February 1969), NA, RG 112, Box 88, Folder: USARV-Americal Division 1960–69.

56. Chas. R. Webb Jr., "Medical Considerations in Internal Defense and Development," *Military Medicine* 133 (May 1968): 395.

57. Billy Akers, MSG, MHIA, AMEDD Oral History Files, Box 1, File 228-01.

58. David P. Allred, Capt., MC, Medical Service Activities Report, 1st Battalion, 46th Infantry, 198th Infantry Brigade (1 January–31 December 1968), NA, RG 112, Box 88, Folder: Americal Division.

59. George F. Brockman, "Medcap to Phou My," *Kentucky Medical Association Journal* 64 (February 1966): 148.

60. Cable 53294 Westmoreland to Admiral Sharp (CINCPAC), Assessment Report (3 August 1967), 3–4, LBJ Library, Collection: NSF, Komer-Leonhart Files, Container 15, Folder: MEMOS—The President 1967.

61. 1/46 198th Infantry Brigade, Army Medical Services Report (28 February 1966), 148.

62. Richard B. Austin, III, (12 June 1969) MHIA, AMEDD Oral History Files, Box 2, File 228-01.

63. Dr. David McK. Rioch, "Summary of Observations and Conclusions of Visit 21 March–9 April 1964," 3, NA, RG 319, Box 38, Folder: #3 History Backup, 17 Feb–30 Apr 1964, Folder 500.

64. Bishop, "Medical Support of Stability Operations," 22.

65. Spurgeon Neel, "The Medical Role in Army Stability Operations," *Military Medicine* 132 (August 1967): 607.

66. Neel, "The Medical Role in Army Stability Operations," 607; William E. Burkhalter, ed., *Surgery in Vietnam: Orthopedic Surgery* (Washington, D.C.: Office of the Surgeon General and Center of Military History, 1994), 16–17.

67. H. E. Leventhal, Medical Civic Action Program Report (29 December to 15 July 1967), Naval BUMED Vietnam Files, Folder: Code 18.

68. "Gaining Confidence," News Release No. 2913 (8 September 1969), Combat Information Bureau III Marine Amphibious Force, Naval BUMED Vietnam File, Folder: Newspaper Clippings and News Releases.

69. Ernest Feigenbaum, End-of-Tour Report (1 May 1967), NA, RG 319, Box 23, Folder: Medical Practice-Vietnam.

70. ADPH Concurrence with Fiegnebaum End-of-Tour Report (3 May 1967), NA, RG 319, Box 23, Folder: Medical Practice-Vietnam.

71. Bishop, "Medical Support of Stability Operations," 34.

72. Sheedy, "Problems Facing Medical Personnel in Counterinsurgency Programs in Southeast Asia," 5–6.

73. Robert W. Komer, "Impact of Pacification on Insurgency in South Vietnam," *Journal of International Affairs* 25 (1971): 59.

74. Ibid., 69.

75. Many authors have addressed aspects of the U.S. attempt to fight a limited well-confined war, while the North Vietnamese intended to fight for as long as it took to win, using whatever means were available. This aspect of the war is addressed by David Callahan, *Unwinnable Wars* (New York: Hill and Wang, 1997); Jamieson, *Understanding Vietnam*; Jeffrey Kimbal, *Nixon's Vietnam War* (Lawrence: University of Kansas Press, 1998); Micheal Lind, *Vietnam: The Necessary War* (New York: The Free Press, 1999); Fredrik Logevall, *Choosing War* (Berkeley and Los Angeles: University of California Press, 1999); and Lewis Sorley, *A Better War* (New York: Harcourt Brace and Company, 1999); David M. Barrett, *Uncertain Warriors: Lyndon Johnson and His Vietnam Advisors* (Lawrence: University of Kansas Press, 1993).

76. M. D. Thomas, Briefing: Vietnamization of Medical Services (2–11 October 1972), Office of the Command Surgeon, NA, RG 319, Box 33, Folder: Briefing on RVNAF med svc 1972.

77. Craddock, "United States Medical Programs in South Vietnam," 187.

78. Fisher, *Dr. America,*" 192.

79. Stanley Allison, MHIA, AMEDD Oral History Files Box 1, 228-01.

Chapter Six: Evaluation of the Programs as a Policy Tool

1. "Some Factors that Influence the Rural Health Program in Vietnam," MAAG Vietnam 1963, 8, NA, RG 319, Box 33, Folder: MAAG, USOM Vietnam 1963/2 USAID.

2. "A Viet Cong force entered the hamlet [Ben Cau] and destroyed building materials that had been placed on a school construction site." Memo for COMUSMACV, Advisory Team 90 Tay Ninh, Current Province Situation 8 May 1964, NA, RG 319, Box 38, Folder: #5 History Backup, 6 May–30 May 1964.

3. 2nd Battalion, 14th Infantry, 25th Division, Army Medical Service Activities Report (7 February 1970), NA, RG 112, Box 78, Folder: USARV–2nd Battalion, 14th Infantry, 25th Division 1960–69.

4. USARV–2nd Battalion, 22nd Infantry, Annual Medical Service Activities Report (1 February 1968), 12, NA, RG 112, Box 78, Folder: USARV–2nd Battalion, 22nd Infantry 1960–69.

5. "Medical Civic Action Program (MEDCAP)," MACV Army Medical Service Activities Report (1964), NA, RG 112, Box 83, Folder: USARV–Military Assistance Command.

6. Chan Cochran, "The Americans who Cried," Navy News Release No. 96F-68 (31 October 1968), Naval BUMED Files, Folder: Newspaper Clippings and News Releases.

7. Spurgeon H. Neel Jr., *Vietnam Studies: Medical Support of the U.S. Army in Vietnam 1965–1970* (Washington, D.C.: Department of the Army, 1991), 180.

8. Westmoreland, *A Soldier Reports,* 349.

9. Ibid., 350.

10. Spurgeon H. Neel Jr., MHIA, Senior Officers Oral History Program, Project 85-D: 160.

11. Gene V. Aaby, MHIA, AMEDDS Oral History File 206-02.1.

12. Neel Papers, MHIA, Senior Officers Oral History Program: 160–61.

13. James W. Kirkpatrick, "Military Medicine in Low Intensity Conflict: A Strategic Analysis," MHIA, Student paper A-DA 233 562 (5 April 1991), 2–3.

14. "AMEDD Aspects of Stability Operations (U)," Department of the Army, Office of the Surgeon General (September 1966), iii, NA, RG 319, Box 31, Folder: AMEDD Aspects of Stability Operations, Jun 67.

15. Ibid., 8.

16. Ibid., 10.

17. Kirkpatrick, "Military Medicine in Low Intensity Conflict," 4–5.

18. Corpsmen as well as doctors and nurses viewed MEDCAP activities as a welcome relief from the tedium of base camp duties. Evans and Sasser, *Doc,* 24–27.

19. Cable JCS 6339-66 from Wheeler to Sharp (CINCPAC) and Westmoreland, NA, RG 319, Box 13, Folder: Message Files COMUSMACV, 1 Oct–31 Dec 1966, Folder 363 [2 of 2]

20. Gen. Spurgeon Neel (retired), interview by author, telephone interview, 15 April 1998.

21. Brig. Gen. David E. Thomas, USARV surgeon, NA, RG 319, Box 39, Folder: Interview with BG Thomas, 12.

22. Ibid., 3.

23. "Some Factors that Influence the Rural Health Program in Vietnam," MAAG Vietnam 1963, 4, NA, RG 319, Box 33, Folder: MAAG, USOM Vietnam 1963/2 USAID.

24. Col. Spurgeon Neel, "U.S. Army Medical Civil Assistance in Viet Nam," 4, NA, RG 112, Box 89, Folder: Medical Care-Medical Civil Action Program (MED CAP).

25. "Command Emphasis on Revolutionary Development/Civic Action Programs," HQ USMACV (22 October 1966) 1, NA, RG 319, Box 28, Folder: #10 History Files 18-29 Oct 1966, Folder 466; Glick, "Military Civic Action," 67.

26. William C. Westmoreland, "Message to All Officers and Men, USMACV (20 June 1964), NA, RG 319, Box 1, Folder: 3 COMUSMACV Public Statements.

27. MSG, Westmoreland MAH794 to Sharp 311050Z Aug 67, Section 5, 3–4, LBJ Library, NSF, Komer-Leonhart File, Container 15, Folder: MEMOS-The President 1967.

28. 85th Evacuation Hospital Newsletter (Jan.–March 1967) 10, NA, RG 112, Box 89.

29. Colonel Carns (MC) served as an infantry platoon leader in Vietnam and as command surgeon, U.S. Southern Command in Panama. Lieutenant Colonel Huebner was with the Directorate of Combat Developments, U.S. Army Academy of Health Sciences, Ft. Sam Houston, Texas. Edwin H.J. Carns and Michael F. Heubner, "Medical Strategy," *Military Review* 69 (February 1989): 37.

30. "I find it unacceptable to draft physicians to serve in this most unpopular war for purposes other than providing medical support for the fighting troops. When a physician is forced by the military to serve in Vietnam, his

primary role is that of providing care for the fighting men. He is not there to carry out a type of Peace Corps work. He is not there to provide medical care for the citizens of another country." Barry S. Levy and Victor W. Sidel., eds., *War and Public Health* (New York: Oxford University Press, 1997), 286. Kirkpatrick, "Military Medicine in Low Intensity Conflict," 16. Donald H. Kuiper, MD, Letter to the Editor "Civilian Casualties in Vietnam," *Annals of Internal Medicine* 75 (August 1971) 324.

31. Howard Levy, "The Military Medicinemen," in John Ehrenreich, ed., *The Cultural Crisis of Modern Medicine* (New York: Monthly Review Press, 1978), 287–300.

32. Richard A. Falk, Gabriel Kolko, and Robert J. Lifton, eds., *Crimes of War* (New York: Vintage Books, Random House, 1971), 434–38.

33. Spurgeon H. Neel Jr. Papers, MHIA, Oral History Collection, 1: 60–67.

34. Greenhut, "I Have Your Wounded," 7.

35. Neel Papers, Oral History Collection, 160.

36. Anderson, "The Field Experience of a Medical Civic Action Team in South Viet Nam," 1056.

37. Glick, "Military Civic Action," 69.

38. James K. Pope (Lt. Col., MC), "Strategic Role of Military Medicine in Developing Countries," MHIA, Student Paper AD-E 750 501 (8 April 1966), 61.

39. U.S. Navy News Release #189-72 (19 February 1972), Naval BUMED Files, Folder: Newspaper Clippings and News Releases.

40. Lieutenant Colonel Taylor served with the Military Public Health Assistance Program in South Vietnam. James A. Taylor, "Military Medicine's Expanding Role in Low-Intensity Conflict," *Military Medicine* (April 1985): 33.

41. 2nd Battalion, 3rd Infantry Medical Service Activities Report (1967), NA, RG 112, Box 79, Folder: USARV-2nd Battalion 3rd Infantry 1960–69.

42. Robin N. Montgomery, "Military Civic Action and Counterinsurgency: The Birth of a Policy" (Ph.D. diss., University of Oklahoma, 1971), 41.

43. "Military Civic Action Teams (MEDCAP)," (15 February 1967) USAID Activity Nr. Project 352.3, NA, RG 112, Box 90, Folder: Historians Source Files Medical Civic Action Program 1965–67.

44. For a more complete breakdown of expenditures and allotments, see Appendix C.

45. Carl E. Bartecchi, *Soc Trang* (Boulder, Colo.: Rocky Mountain Guild, 1980), 103.

46. Westmoreland to Sharp, MAC Message 5740 (8 July 1966), Westmoreland Papers, MHIA, Box 27, Folder: History File 7, May 26 to July 16, 1966.

47. Col. Marvin A. Ware, chief, supply division, office of the Surgeon Gen-

eral, letter (11 January 1969), NA, RG 112, Box 1, Folder: Black-marketing Pharmaceuticals 1970–71.

48. Brig. Gen. James L. Collins Jr., special assistant to COMUSMACV, Memorandum for the Record of Nha Trang Conference (24 October 1965), NA, RG 319, Box 26, Folder: #1 History File, 19 Aug–24 Oct 1965, Folder 458.

49. Lt. Col. John Bullard (MSC), U.S. Civil Assistance Programs in SVN Fact Sheet (29 April 1971) 2, MHI-VNR, Folder: 2012 01.

50. Glick, "Military Civic Action," 70.

51. Hoyt R. Livingston and Francis M. Watson Jr., "Civic Action: Purpose and Pitfalls," *Military Review* 47 (December 1967): 25.

52. Bishop, "Medical Support of Stability Operations," 13–14.

53. Gen. William C. Westmoreland, "Opening Remarks for 8th Quarterly Psywar/CA Conference," (6 August 1964), NA, RG 319, Box 39, Folder: #7 History Backup, 27 July–31 Aug 1964, Folder 504.

54. "Report of Visit by Dept. of Army Staff Team to the Republic of Vietnam, 28 March–4 April 1964," 17, CMH, Drawer: HRC Geog V. Vietnam, Folder: 319.1 Army Staff Visit, 28 Mar–4 April 1964.

55. General Westmoreland, *Report on the War in Vietnam,* Military History Branch, MACV (30 June 1968), 270, CMH, Drawer: Geog V. Vietnam 319.1 to 319.1, Folder: Report on the War in V.N., Gen. W. C. Westmoreland.

56. Office of the Surgeon, MACV, Medical Activities Report (1965), NA, RG 112, Box 91, Folder: USARV-MAAG 1960–69.

57. "Message from the Surgeon General (DA TB 8-19, TSG, Oct 66)" contained in "Medical Newsletter," HQ U.S. Army John F. Kennedy Center for Special Warfare (Airborne), Ft. Bragg, N.C. (1 February 1967), NA, RG 319, Box 32, Folder: Surgeon's Newsletter.

58. Livingston and Watson, "Civic Action: Purpose and Pitfalls," 23.

59. Baker, "Medical Assistance to the Vietnamese," 10.

60. Bobby N. Huntington, 58th Medical Battalion Army Medical Service Activities Report (1968), 12, NA, RG 112, Box 80, Folder: USARV-Battalions-58th Medical 1960–69.

61. "Civilian Medical Program for Vietnam (Follow-up Investigation)," Thirty-fifth Report (No. 91-1584) House of Representatives, 91st Congress, 2nd Session (Washington, DC: Government Printing Office), 8 October 1970, 3–17.

62. Office of the Surgeon General, Memorandum No. 381-2 (30 April 1974), NA, RG 319, Box 23, Folder: Medical Intelligence.

63. SGO Office Order No. 87 (18 April 1941); Gaylor W. Anderson, "Medical Intelligence," chap. 5 in Ebbe C. Hoff, ed., *Preventive Medicine in World War II* (Washington, D.C.: Office of the Surgeon General, 1969), 3.

64. Ibid., 4.

65. "Medical Intelligence," FM 8-30 (1951), Medical Field Service School, Brooke Army Medical Center, Fort Sam Houston, Tex.

66. Anderson, "Medical Intelligence," 252, 337.

67. 2nd Battalion, 3rd Infantry, Medical Service Activities Report (1967), NA, RG 112, Box 79, Folder: USARV-2nd Battalion, 3rd Infantry 1960–69.

68. "Civic Action Newsletter #10," (10 July 1967), NA, RG 472, Box 2, Folder: 201-46 MEDCAP 1967.

69. SGM Patsy Angelone, End of Tour Interview (7 November 1975) 19, NA, RG 319, Box 36, Folder: Angelone, Patsy SGM, 2nd Bn, 5th SFG.

70. James R. Lay, "How Tactical Units of the U.S. Army in Vietnam Can Get the Most out of Civic Action with the Minimum Cost and Expenditure of Resources," MHIA, Student Paper 680 972 (17 January 1968), 2.

71. Irving, "The 'Other War'?" 25–26.

72. Webb, "Medical Considerations in Internal Defense and Development," 393.

73. Anderson, "Medical Intelligence," 393.

74. Fred G. Weyand, "Winning the People in Hau Nghia Province," *Army* 17 (January 1967): 55.

75. 25th Division Assistant Chief of Staff, G-2, Intelligence Summaries, NA, RG 472, Boxes 1 through 9, Folders by the Month [especially Box 4, Folder: 16–30 April 1968].

76. 1st Cavalry Division Assistant Chief of Staff G-2 Supplemental Intelligence Reports G-2, NA, RG 472, USARV 1st Cavalry Division, Box 1; 1st Infantry Division Assistant Chief of Staff Intelligence Reports G-2, NA, RG 472, USARV 1st Infantry Division, Box 1.

77. Stolfi, *U.S. Marine Corps Civic Action Efforts in Vietnam March 1965–March 1966,* 31.

78. Cornelius D. Sullivan et al., *The Vietnam War: Its Conduct and Higher Direction* (Washington, D.C.: Center for Strategic Studies, Georgetown University, 1968), 90.

79. General Khanh was commander in II Corps in 1963, active in the coup against President Ngo Dinh Diem, and subsequently became premier of South Vietnam until he was ousted in February 1965. Memorandum for the Record, meeting between General Westmoreland and General Khanh (8 December 1964), NA, RG 319, Box 39, Folder: #11 History Backup, 7 Dec–31 Dec 1964, Folder 509.

80. Robin N. Montgomery, "Military Civic Action and Counterinsurgency: The Birth of a Policy" (Ph.D. diss., University of Oklahoma, 1971), 136–45.

81. President Lyndon B. Johnson News Conference (5 July 1966), *Selected Statements on Vietnam by DoD and Other Administrative Officials July 1–December 31, 1966,* prepared by Research and Analysis Division SAF-AAR (10 April 1967). Military History Institute Library.

82. Debriefing Report (RCS-SCFOR-74) BG Glenn J. Collins for 11 July 1967–1 August 1967 (1 August 1967), NA, RG 112, Box 1.

83. John A. Sheedy (Col., MC), "Medical Implications of Wars of Liberation in Southeast Asia," MHIA, Student Paper AD-B 217 097 (6 April 1966), 6.

84. Pope, "Strategic Role of Military Medicine in Developing Nations," 11, 69–70.

85. Sheedy, "Medical Implications of Wars of Liberation," 2.

86. Robert W. Komer, Statements upon returning from Vietnam Revolutionary Development Program (2 July 1966), *Selected Statements on Vietnam by DoD and Other Administrative Officials July 1–December 31, 1966,* prepared by Research and Analysis Division SAF-AAR (10 April 1967), Military History Institute Library.

87. Ambassador Robert Komer, interview by author, telephone interview, 17 February 1996.

88. Neel, *Medical Support of the U.S. Army in Vietnam,* 164.

89. Bishop, "Medical Support of Stability Operations," 13.

90. Jenkins, "Medical Civic Action Programs," 10.

91. Ibid., 10–11.

92. Ibid., 11.

93. Bishop, "Medical Support of Stability Operations," 23.

94. Mitchell, "Medic as an Instrument of National Policy," 2.

95. William C. Holmberg, "Civic Action," *Marine Corps Gazette* 50 (June 1966): 28.

96. Matthew S. Klimow, "Moral *versus* Practical: The Future of US Armed Humanitarian Intervention," U.S. Army War College Senior Service Fellows Program Paper A-DA 314 726 (Center for International Relations, Queens University, Kinston, Ont., Canada, 1996), 92.

97. Kirkpatrick, "Military Medicine in Low Intensity Conflict," 8–9.

98. Ian L. Natkin, "The Role of Health Services in support of the Theater Campaign Plan," MHIA, Student Paper AD-A 208 619 (30 March 1989), 4.

99. Jenkins, "Medical Civic Action Programs," 44.

100. Kirkpatrick, "Military Medicine in Low Intensity Conflict," 9.

101. Ibid., 17.

102. Bishop, "Medical Support of Stability Operations," iii.

103. As far back as the Philippine Insurrection "The Army realized that fre-

quent rotations harmed its pacification efforts." Birtle, *U.S. Army counterinsurgency and Contingency Operations and Doctrine 1860–1941,* 162–63.

104. David V. Brown, "Civilian Public Health Programs in Vietnam 1966–1970—A Review," Medical Survey Vietnam–1970, Report No. B-11, NA, RG 319, Box 38, Folder: USAID Medical Programs.

105. Jenkins, "Medical Civic Action Programs," 12, 43.

106. Brian M. Jenkins, "The Unchangeable War," RM-6278-ARPA (Santa Monica, Calif.: Rand Corporation Paper, November 1970), 1.

107. David Halberstam, "Return to Vietnam," *Harper's Magazine* 235 (December 1967): 51.

108. Commentary by Stanley Karnow, "Some Lessons and Non-Lessons of Vietnam," 23.

109. Ben Kiernan, "Review Article: The Vietnam War: Alternative Endings," *American Historical Review* 97 (October 1992): 1136–37.

110. Marilyn B. Young, *The Vietnam Wars 1945–1990* (New York: Harper Collins, 1991), 167.

111. Hans J. Morgenthau, "Bundy's Doctrine of War without End," *The New Republic* 159 (2 November 1968): 19.

112. Bernard B. Fall, "Indochina: The Last Year of the War, the Navarre Plan," *Military Review* 34 (December 1954): 56.

113. Haakon Ragde, "Medicine in Vietnam," letter to the editor, *Journal of the American Medical Association* 215 (March 29, 1971): 2114.

114. Taylor and Fields, "Health Care as an Instrument of Foreign Policy," 25.

115. Westmoreland, *Report on the War in Vietnam (as of 30 June 1968) Section II,* (USMACV, 1968), 239.

Chapter Seven: Conclusions

1. Cramblet, "U.S. Medical Imperatives for Low Intensity Conflict," 7.

2. Comments made by General Moshe Dayan, NA, RG 319, Box 34, Folder: #32 History File, 1–31 May 1968, Folder 488.

3. HQ MAAG, "Lessons Learned Number 30: Psychological Warfare and Civic Action Operations," (17 August 1963) 6, NA, RG 319, Box 37, Folder: #1 History Backup, 30 March 1962–Nov 1963, Folder 48-98 [2 of 2].

4. Sorley, *A Better War,* 216.

5. Eduard Mark, "Revolution by Degrees: Stalin=National-Front Strategy for Europe, 1941–1947," Working paper No. 31 (February 2001) Cold War International History Project, Woodrow Wilson International Center for Scholars, Washington, D.C.

6. Spurgeon H. Neel Jr., MHIA, Senior Officers Oral History Program, Project 85-D, 1: 162.

7. HQ USMACV Monthly Evaluation Report (July 1965), 6, MHI-VNR.

8. I Field Force, Army Medical Service Activities Report (8 February 1967), 9, NA, RG 112, Box 90, Folder: USARV-I Field Force 1960–69.

9. Sorley, *A Better War.*

10. "On at least one occasion, the civic action program enabled USAF and VNAF officials to thwart a planned mortar attack on Binh Thuy AB in the fall of 1966." Carl Berger, ed., *The United States Air Force in Southeast Asia, 1961–1973: An Illustrated Account* (Washington, D.C.: Office of Air Force History, 1984), 289.

11. David V. Brown, Medical Survey Vietnam—1970 Report No. B-11, p. 8, NA, RG 319, Box 38, Folder: USAID Medical Programs.

12. Comments of General Thang at a Revolutionary Development Meeting, II Corps (27 May 1968), NA, RG 319, Box 34, Folder: #32 History File, 1–31 May 1968, Folder 488 [3 of 3].

13. Robert L. Burke, "Military Civic Action," *Military Review* 44 (October 1964): 68.

14. Comments Made by General Moshe Dayan, NA, RG 319, Box 34, Folder: #32 History File, 1–31 May 1968, Folder 488.

15. Nha Trang Conference (24 October 1965), NA, RG 319, Box 34, Folder: #1 History File, 19 Aug–24 Oct 1965, Folder 458.

16. Allan W. Kenner (Col., SF), "Korea to Kalimantan and Beyond: The Employment of United States Army Forces in Military Civic Action in the Pacific Command Area of Responsibility," MHIA, Student Paper AD-A 223 348 (9 April 1990), 53.

17. Progress Report (30 December 1967), Children's Medical Relief International, Inc., LBJ Library, NSF, Komer-Leonhart File, Box 14, Folder: Medical Relief [1 of 2].

18. Medical Appraisal Team Report (20 September 1967), LBJ Library, NSF, Komer-Leonhart File, Container #14, Folder: Medical Relief [1 of 2].

19. Jenkins, "Medical Civic Action Programs," 44.

20. Dick Wilson, "The American Quarter-Century in Asia," *Foreign Affairs* 51 (July 1973): 830.

21. Kenner, "Korea to Kalimantan and Beyond," 55.

22. Arthur M. Ahern, "Medicine in Internal Defense," *Military Review* 47 (September 1967): 69.

23. "Medical Aspects of Counterinsurgency," Speech Ft. Bragg, NC (15 April 1965), MHIA, Leonard D. Heaton Papers, Box 10, Book 3, Folder: Speech File 1965.

24. Remarks Pan-Pacific Surgical Association, Honolulu, HI (20 September 1966), MHIA, Leonard D. Heaton Papers, Box 10.

25. Address to 95th Annual Meeting of West Virginia State Medical Association (23 Aug 1962), MHIA, Leonard D. Heaton Papers, Box 9, Book #2.

26. William A. Boyson, "Medico-Military Contribution to Nation Building," MHIA, Student Paper 670 172 (1967), 4.

27. Barry N. Totten (Lt. Col., USA), "The Army's Role in Humanitarian Assistance, Challenges Now and in the Future," MHIA, Student Paper AD-A 308 633 (15 April 1996), 1.

28. Pope, "Strategic Role of Military Medicine in Developing Nations," 52.

29. "Once begun, military civic action may be very difficult to end . . . There are psychological problems in civic action. Some civilians and soldiers consider it beyond the proper pale of the military. Can troops really be shuttled back and forth, easily and quickly, between civic action and combat?" Glick, "Military Civic Action," 68.

30. Seth Cropsey, "The Hard Truth about 'Soft Missions,'" *The Wall Street Journal,* 19 January 1993, A-14.

31. Robert G. Claypool (Col., MC), "Military Medicine as an Instrument of Power: An Overview and Assessment," MHIA, Student Paper AD-A 209 270 (31 March 1989), 23.

32. In the early 1960s, South Vietnam had only 1,400 physicians, 1,000 of whom were in their army. Even though many physicians serving in the army also had civilian practices, there were only four hundred nonmilitary physicians to care for 16 million civilians. Almost all nonmilitary physicians were located in the major cities, mainly Saigon, Da Nang, and Hué. Lee, "Surgical Care of Civilians in Viet Nam," 811–12. There was also a severe shortage of nurses, most of whom were men and drafted into the military. Fiedler, "Medical Care in Vietnam," 20–22; Charles R. Webb Jr., Medical Newsletter, Office of the Surgeon, Ft. Bragg, N.C. (1 June 1967) 4, NA, RG 319, Box 32, Folder: Surgeon's Newsletter.

33. Birtle, *U.S. Army Counterinsurgency and Contingency Operations Doctrine 1860–1941,* 124–25.

34. "The major difficulty that has been encountered is the relative failure of the Vietnamese civil or military services to become identified with providing such medical aid to the people, and that the local populations are left with the impression that it is only the Americans that render such care and not their own government. Thus the present program promises to have little sustaining or long range effect in so far as maintaining or improving regard for the Vietnamese government." *Report of Military Medical Research Pro-*

gram Survey Group 17 July 1962–11 January 1963, NA, RG 112, Medical R & D in S.E. Asia and Vietnam Box 92, Folder E1015.

35. Ambassador Maxwell Taylor, Mission Council Briefing (14 September 1964), NA, RG 319, Box 39, Folder: #10 History Backup, 14 Nov–7 Dec 1967, Folder 507.

Appendix A: Patients Treated in MEDCAP

1. For the period 1963 through 1965, there were 29 teams with 127 personnel. MACV Command Overview from Command Surgeon to Military History Branch, March 1972, NA, RG 319 Box 33, Folder: MACV-Surgeon-Cmd Overview for 1971.

2. For 1966 through 1967, MEDCAP activities were performed by RVNAF, U.S., and FWMAF units; for the period 1968 through 1971 reports are for United States and FWMAF only, which accounts for the sharp reduction in MEDCAP treatments reported; 1971 figures are for six months.

Appendix C: Expenditures

1. AID Memorandum for McGeorge Bundy, The White House (30 October 1962), Subject: National Security Action Memorandum 119, NA, RG 319 Civic Action Planning Files, 1960–65 Box 1, Folder: Military Civic Action.

2. Some Factors That Influence the Rural Health Program in Vietnam, MAAG Vietnam 1963, NA, RG 319, Box 33, Folder: MAAG, USOM Vietnam 1963/2 USAID.

3. J5 Memorandum: Intensification of Civic Action Programs in Republic of Vietnam (30 September 1963), NA, RG 319, Box 38, Folder: #2 History Backup, Jan 64–4 Feb 1964, Folder 499.

4. C. L. Jones, Information Brief, Subject: Civic Action—South Vietnam (n.d.), NA, RG 319, Box 8, Information Book for C of S U.S. Army Visit to Far East and Pacific, 2–18 Dec 1964.

5. Bishop, "Medical Support of Stability Operations," 12.

6. USMACV, Army Medical Service Activities Report (1964), NA, RG 112, Box 83, Folder: USARV-Military Assistance Command.

7. Memorandum of Understanding Between the DOA and AID (November 1966), NA, RG 472, HQ, U.S. Army Vietnam, Surgeon Section, Plans and Operations Division Box 2, Folder: 201-46 MEDCAP 1967.

8. William C. Westmoreland Papers, MHIA, Box 27, Folder: History File 7, May 26–July 16, 1966.

9. U.S.G. Sharp and W. C. Westmoreland, "Report on the War in Vietnam (as of 30 June 1968), 239, Military History Institute Library.

10. William H. Moncreif Jr., "The Provincial Health Program in the Republic of Vietnam," *USARV Medical Bulletin* 2 (Jan–Feb 1967): 39.

11. Program Status Report—Month of October 1967 (15 November 1967), NA, RG 112, Box 60, Folder: #3 Health—Civilians Assistance.

12. "Civilian Medical Program for Vietnam," House Report No. 91-1584, 91st Congress, 2nd Session, Committee on Government Operations, (Washington, D.C.: Government Printing Office, 1970), 17.

13. Report to Subcommittee to Investigate Problems Connected with Refugees and Escapees Committee on the Judiciary, U.S. Senate, by the comptroller general of the United States (9 November 1970), 2, NA, RG 319, Box 33, Folder: Civilian Health and War Related Casualty Programs (5).

14. Subcommittee Report, ibid., 13.

15. Ibid.

16. Ibid., 14.

17. Statement of Ambassador William E. Colby to Subcommittee on Refugees and Escapees of the Senate Committee on the Judiciary (21 April 1971), NA, RG 319, Box 33, Folder: Ambassador Colby (6).

18. MACMD Fact Sheet: Joint Medical Construction Program in Vietnam (21 May 1968), NA, RG 319, Box 40, Folder: Fact Book—COMUSMACV, Folder 516.

19. AID/DID Realignment Estimates, NA, RG 112, Records of the Office of the Surgeon General (Army), Box 90, Folder: Medical Civic Action Program 1965–67.

20. AID/DOD Project Definition Summary Sheet, Medicines for Military Civic Action Teams, NA, RG 112, Box 90, Folder: 228-02 Medical Civic Action Program 1965–67.

21. AID/DOD Program Realignments for Operations in Vietnam, Joint MACV/USAIDV Message 14091 (29 April 1967), NA, RG 472, HQ U.S. Army Vietnam, Surgeon Section, Plans and Operations Division Box 2, Folder: 201-46 MEDCAP 1967.

22. MACMD Fact Sheet (21 May 1968): Civilian War Casualty Program, NA, RG 319, Box 40, Folder: Fact Book—COMUSMACV, Folder 516.

23. Project Status and Accomplishment Report USAID/Vietnam (30 January 1970), Project, Medical Care, Number: 730-11-530-347, NA, RG 112, Box 60, Folder: Subject Files, 1960–69.

24. Robert Bernstein, Medical Service in the Republic of Vietnam January 1970–April 1972, Office of the Command Surgeon, HQ MACV, MHIA, AMEDDS Oral History Collection.

25. Memorandum of Understanding between the DOA and AID (25 May 1967), MHI-VNR, Folder: AID/DOD Realignment Program.

26. Young, *The Vietnam Wars 1945–1990,* 210.

27. *Statistical Abstract of the United States* (1970), 247.

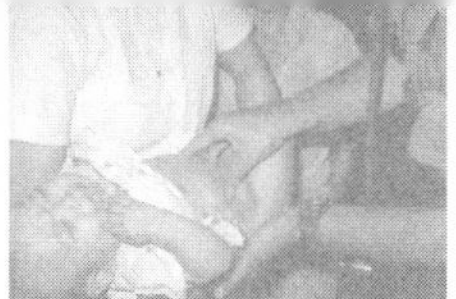

Glossary

AFAK: Armed Forces Assistance to Korea
AGHD: Administration General for Health Development
AID: Agency for International Development
AMEDD: Army Medical Department
AMEDS: Army Medical Service
APC: Armed personnel carriers
ARVN: Army, Republic of Vietnam
ASF: Army Service Forces
CAP: Combined Action Platoon
CARE: Cooperative for American Relief Everywhere
CHO: Chief Health Officer (GVN)
CIA: Central Intelligence Agency
CIDG: Civilian Irregular Defense Group
CINCPAC: Commander in Chief, Pacific (the direct line of command over COMUSMACV)
CJCS: Chairman, Joint Chiefs of Staff
COMUSMACV: Commander, USMACV
CONUS: Continental United States
CORDS: Civil Operations, Revolutionary Development Support
CWCP: Civilian War Casualty Program
DA: Department of Army
DENTCAP: Dental Civic Action Program
DIA: Defense Intelligence Agency

DMZ: Demilitarized Zone (between North and South Vietnam)
DOD: Department of Defense
EDCOR: Economic Development Corps Program
EMS: Emergency Medical Services
FWMAF: Free World Military Assistance Forces
GAO: Government Accounting Office
GVN: Government of Vietnam or the Republic of Vietnam
JU: Joint Utilization Program
JUSPAO: Joint U.S. Public Affairs Office
LIC: Low Intensity Conflict
LSM: Landing Ship Medical
MAAG: Military Assistance Advisory Group
MAC: Military Assistance Command
MACV: Military Assistance Command, Vietnam
MAF: Marine Amphibious Force (III MAF)
MAP: Military Assistance Program
MASH: Mobile Army Surgical Hospital
MASP: Military Assistance Service-support Program
MC: Medical Corps
MEDCAP: Medical Civic Action Program
MHSWR: Ministry of Health, Social Welfare and Refugees (GVN)
MI: Military Intelligence
MIIA: Medical Intelligence and Information Agency
MILPHAP: Military Provincial Hospital Augmentation Program, later changed to Military Provincial Health Program
MOD: (Vietnamese) Ministry of Defense
MOH: (Vietnamese) Ministry of Health
MORD: Ministry of Revolutionary Development (GVN)
MPCC: Medical Policy Coordinating Committee of U.S. Mission Council
MSC: Medical Service Corps
MUST: Medical Unit, Self-Contained, Transportable
NAVFORV: Naval Force, Vietnam
NGO: Nongovernmental organizations

Glossary

NLF: National Liberation Front
NSA: Naval Support Activity
NSAM: National Security Action Memorandum
NVA: North Vietnamese Army
OCO: Office of Civil Operations
OER: Officer Efficiency Reports
OMI: *Otdel Myezhdunarodnoi Informatzii*
OSA: Office of the Special Assistant (a CIA operative)
OSS: Office of Strategic Services
PAVN: People's Army of Vietnam (North Vietnam)
PF: Popular Forces
PHAP: Provincial Health Assistance Project
PHILCAGV: Philippine Civic Action Group, Vietnam
Philcon V: Philippine Contingent to Vietnam
POW: Prisoner of war
Project HOPE: Health Opportunities for People Everywhere
PROVN: Program for the Pacification and Long-Term Development of South Vietnam
Psyops: Psychological operations
RD: Revolutionary Development
RF: Regional Forces
ROK: Republic of Korea
RVN: Republic of Vietnam (South Vietnam)
RVNAF: Republic of Vietnam Armed Forces
SF: Special Forces
TAOC: Tactical Area of Command
TAOR: Tactical Area of Operational Responsibility
TDY: Temporary duty orders
III MAF: III Marine Amphibious Force
USAID: United States Agency for International Development
USARPAC: U.S. Army, Pacific
USARV: United States Army, Vietnam
USIA: United States Information Agency
USIS: United States Information Service

USMC: United States Marine Corps
USOM: United States Overseas Mission
USPHS: United States Public Health Service
USUHS: Uniformed Services University of the Health Sciences
VC: Viet Cong
VN: Vietnam
VPVN: Volunteer Physicians for Vietnam
WRAIR: Walter Reed Army Institute of Research

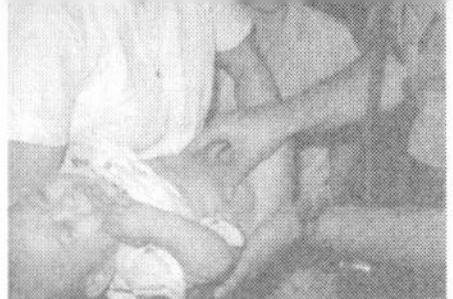

Bibliographic Essay

The literature regarding military medicine is voluminous. Even limiting a review to works pertaining to the United States and its forces abroad encompasses a vast number of volumes.

Medical care in the Civil War is discussed in the two companion pieces, George W. Adams, *Doctors in Blue: The Medical History of the Union Army in the Civil War* (New York: Henry Schuman, 1952) and H. H. Cunningham, *Doctors in Gray: The Confederate Medical Service* (Baton Rouge: Louisiana State University Press, 1960). Other works on this topic include William Q. Maxwell, *Lincoln's Fifth Wheel* (New York: Longmans, Green & Co., 1956); and Harold E. Straubing, *In Hospital and Camp: The Civil War through the Eyes of Its Doctors and Nurses* (Harrisburg, Pa.: Stackpole Books, 1993).

The Spanish-American War era at the end of the nineteenth century and the subsequent insurrection in the Philippines are focused on by Graham A. Cosmas, *An Army for Empire: The United States Army in the Spanish-American War* (Shippensburg, Pa.: White Mane Publishing, 1994); John M. Gibson, *The Life of General William C. Gorgas;* Nicholas Senn, *Medico-Surgical Aspects of the Spanish American War* (Chicago: American Medical Association, 1900); Warwick Anderson, "Colonial Pathologies: American Medicine in the Philippines, 1898–1921,"

(Ph.D. diss., University of Pennsylvania, 1992); and Mary C. Gillette, *Army Medical Department 1865–1917.*

P. S. Bond and C. F. Martin, *Medical Service in Modern War* (Menasha, Wis.: George Banta, 1920) discuss World War I.

World War II receives extensive attention, including Albert E. Cowdrey, *Fighting for Life: American Military Medicine in World War II* (New York: The Free Press, 1994); the multivolume series by Surgeon General Leonard D. Heaton, *History of the Medical Department of the United States Army in World War II* under the auspices of the Office of the Surgeon General (Washington, D.C.: Department of the Army, 1956–69); George Sharpe, *Brothers Beyond Blood: A Battalion Surgeon in the South Pacific* (Austin: Diamond Books, 1989); and Charles M. Wiltse, *The Medical Department: Medical Service in the Mediterranean and Minor Theaters, United States Army in World War II, The Technical Services* (Washington, D.C.: Office of the Chief of Military History, Department of the Army, 1965).

The often ignored Korean conflict is dealt with by Albert E. Cowdrey, *The Medic's War;* and Crawford W. Sams, *"Medic."*

Many of the "standard" texts dealing with the Vietnam conflict totally disregard the use of medical services to aid the civilians or mention the topic only in passing: George C. Herring, *America's Longest War: The United States and Vietnam, 1950–1975,* Second Edition (New York: Alfred Knopf, 1986); Stanley Karnow, *Vietnam: A History* (New York: Penguin, 1991); Gabriel Kolko, *Anatomy of a War, Vietnam, the United States, and the Modern Historical Experience* (New York: The New Press, 1994); Gunter Lewy, *America in Vietnam* (New York: Oxford University Press, 1978); Robert D. Schulzinger, *A Time for War: The United States and Vietnam, 1941–1975* (New York: Oxford University Press, 1997); Harry G. Summers Jr., *On Strategy: A Critical Analysis of the Vietnam War* (Novato, Calif.: Presidio Press, 1982); and Spencer C. Tucker, *Vietnam* (Lexington: University Press of Kentucky, 1999).

Texts dealing with medical services in the Vietnam War include Spurgeon Neel, *Medical Support of the U.S. Army in Vietnam.* Even works specifically addressing the question of pacification rarely mention medical services other than in passing, as Scoville, *Reorganizing for Pacification Support;* Hunt, *Pacification;* Edward P. Metzner, *More than a Soldier's War: Pacification in Vietnam* (College Station: Texas A&M University Press, 1995), and Charles R. Anderson, *Vietnam: The Other War.*

There are many memoirs and diaries by doctors, nurses, and corpsmen who served in Vietnam. Those by physicians include Carl E. Bartecchi, *Soc Trang: A Vietnamese Odyssey* (Boulder, Colo.: Rocky Mountain Writers Guild, 1980); Wesley G. Byerly Jr., *Nam Doc* (New York: Vantage Press, 1981) and *Trung Ta Bac Si* (Baltimore, Md.: Gateway Press, 1986); Byron E. Holley, *Vietnam 1968–1969, A Battalion Surgeon's Journal* (New York: Ivy Books, 1993); Larry Kammholz, *Moc Hoa: A Vietnam Medical-Military Adventure* (Oshkosh, Wis.: Starboard Publishing, 1989); Andrew Lovy, *Vietnam Diary: October 1967–July 1968* (New York: The Exposition Press, 1970); John Parrish, *12, 20 & 5, A Doctor's Year in Vietnam* (New York: E.P. Dutton & Co., 1972). For information regarding nurses see Jeanne Holm, *Women in the Military: An Unfinished Revolution* (Novato, Calif.: Presidio, 1982); Jan Hornung, *Angles in Vietnam: Women Who Served* (Lincoln, Nebr.: Writers Club Press, 2002); Olga Gruhzit-Hoyt, *A Time Remembered: American Women in the Vietnam War* (Novato, Calif.: Presidio Press, 1999); Elizabeth Norman, *Women at War: The Story of Fifty Military Nurses who Served in Vietnam* (Philadelphia: University of Pennsylvania Press, 1990); Winnie Smith, *America's Daughter Gone to War: On the Front Lines as an Army Nurse in Vietnam* (New York: Pocket Books, 1992); Ron Steinman, *Women in Vietnam, The Oral History* (New York: TV Books, 2000); Lynda Van Devanter, *Home Before Morning: The Story of an Army Nurse in Vietnam* (Amherst: University of Massachusetts Press, 1983, 2001); and Keith Walker, *A Piece of*

My Heart: The Stories of Twenty-six Women Who Served in Vietnam (Novato, Calif.: Presidio Press, 1985). Medics are treated in Craig Roberts, *Combat Medic: Vietnam* (New York: Pocket Books, 1998); and Daniel E. Evans and Charles W. Sasser, *Doc: Platoon Medic.* John Cook discussed the history and development of the helicopter medical evacuation system in *Rescue Under Fire: The Story of Dust Off in Vietnam* (Atglen, Pa.: Schiffer Military/Aviation History, 1998), as did Michael J. Novosel in *Dustoff: The Memoir of an Army Aviator* (New York: Ballantine Books, 1999). Another memoir dealing with medical evacuation is B. W. Miller, *The Newbe* (Florence, Ala.: HiString Records Inc., 1973). These narratives tend to be highly anecdotal and devoid of policy analysis. As is apparent from their titles, they tend to be limited to a restricted perspective, suffering geographically and temporally. They reflect what occurred in one place at one time.

Recent works, many of which originate within the military, give more attention to the use of medicine as an instrument of policy, but all lack a full discussion as well as suggestions for future use: Berry, "Medicine and United States Foreign Policy," 15–17; Claypool, "Military Medicine as an Instrument of Power"; Jenkins, "Medical Civic Action Programs"; Kenner, "Korea to Kalimantan and Beyond"; Mitchell, "Medic as an Instrument of National Policy"; James A. Taylor, "Military Medicine's Expanding Role in Low-Intensity Conflict," *Military Medicine* 65 (April 1985): 26–34. This is also true in the work by U.S. allies, Brendan O'Keefe, *Medicine at War: Medical Aspects of Australia's Involvement in Southeast Asian Conflicts 1950–1972* (St. Leonards, NSW, Australia: Allen & Unwin Pty Ltd., 1994).

The psychological aspects of combat in Vietnam are highlighted in Eric F. Dean Jr., *Shook Over Hell: Post-Traumatic Stress, Vietnam and the Civil War* (Cambridge, Mass.: Harvard University Press, 1997), and Jonathan Shay, *Achilles in Vietnam: Combat Trauma and the Undoing of Character* (New York: Atheneum, 1994).

Some of the "official" histories that touch on these topics include Hal B. Jennings Jr., *A Decade of Progress: The United States Army Medical Department 1959–1969* (Washington, D.C.: Office of the Surgeon General, 1971); Mary T. Sarnecky, *A History of the U.S. Army Nurse Corps* (Philadelphia: University of Pennsylvania Press, 1999); William H. H. Clark, *The History of the United States Army Veterinary Corps in Vietnam 1962–1973* (Roswell, Ga.: W.H. Wolfe Associates, 1992); and Richard V. N. Ginn, *History of the U.S. Army Medical Service Corps.* There is also a series of technical works put out by the Office of the Surgeon General and the Center of Military History, with titles such as *Internal Medicine in Vietnam, General Medicine and Infectious Disease,* or *Skin Diseases in Vietnam 1965–72.* There are similar works for orthopedics, etc.

The medical aspects of the war from the viewpoint of the north are detailed in Nguyen Khac Vien, ed., *North Vietnamese Medicine Faction the Trails of War* (Hanoi: Vietnamese Studies, 1967).

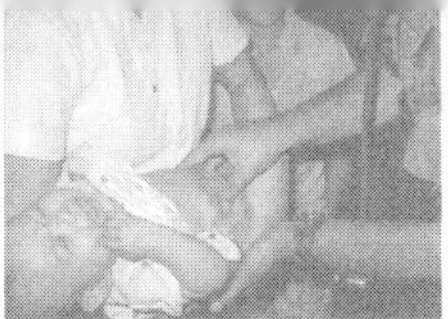

Index

Index

Index

Index

Index

OTHER BOOKS IN THE MODERN SOUTHEAST ASIA SERIES

Vietnam and Beyond: A Diplomat's Cold War Education,
by Robert Hopkins Miller

Window on a War: An Anthropologist in the Vietnam Conflict,
by Gerald C. Hickey

Vietnam Chronicles: The Abrams Tapes, 1968–1972, transcribed and edited by Lewis Sorley